NOTABLE PLANTS IN ETHNOMEDICINE

OF MADHYA PRADESH

NOTABLE PLANTS IN ETHNOMEDICINE

OF MADHYA PRADESH

Dinesh Jadhav

Assistant Professor

Department of Botany

Govt. Arts & Science College, Ratlam (M. P.)

AUTHORSPRESS

Worldwide Circulation through Authorspress Global Network
First Published in 2022
by
Authorspress
Q-2A Hauz Khas Enclave, New Delhi-110 016 (India)
Phone: (0) 9818049852
E-mail: authorspressgroup@gmail.com
Website: www.authorspressbooks.com

Notable Plants in Ethnomedicine of Madhya Pradesh

ISBN 978-93-5529-204-9

Printed in India a Kensington Press

Dedicated to

The Memory of My Grandmother

Late Mrs. ***Kanchan Devi Jadhav***

Acknowledgements

First and foremost I express my deep sense of gratitude and indebtedness to Respected Dr R. L. Mehra, Chairman, Madhya Pradesh Public Service Commission, Indore (M.P.), Respected Dr. Anil K. Goel, Retd Deputy Director, Botanic Garden, National Botanical Research institute (NBRI), Lucknow (Uttar Pradesh), Dr. S. K. Agarwal (Retd Professor, Department of Botany, DBS College, Dehra Dun, Uttarakhand) and Dr R.L.S. Sikarwar (Deendayal Research Institute, Chitrakoot, Satna) for encouragement, keen interest, support and co-operation.

I express my deep sense of gratitude to Respected Shri. J. C. Chauhan, Retd. Prof. and Head, Department of Botany, Govt. Arts and Science College, Ratlam (M. P.), Respected Dr. Sanjay Wate, Principal, Govt. Arts and Science College, Ratlam (M. P.), Respected Dr. Rajkumar Katare, Principal, Govt. Girls Degree College, Ratlam (M. P.), Respected Mrs. Sushma Raj Katare, Professor and Head, Department of Botany, Govt. Girls Degree College, Ratlam (M. P.), Respected Dr. Abhay Pathak, Professor, Govt. Vivekananda Commerce College, Ratlam (M. P.), Respected Dr Bhavana Deshpande, Professor, Department of Mathematics, Govt. Arts and Science College, Ratlam (M. P.) and Respected Shri. Manoj Verma, Professor, Department of English, Govt. College, Satna (M. P.) for encouragement, keen interest, support and valuable co-operation.

Dinesh Jadhav

Preface

Madhya Pradesh is rich in floristic as well as ethnic diversity. It comprises 45 Districts and forest covers 30.9 % of the total area of the state. More than 41 tribal communities resides in or around the forests and depend mainly on forest resources for their daily requirements like food, fodder, fibre, gum, resin, tannin, wood, medicines, dye for ascertaining the ethnobotanical status of the state. Presently, there are a number of ethnobotanical studies in different tribal inhabited localities of Madhya Pradesh are being carried out actively. The book deals with the 266 species of probable Ethnomedicinal potential from tribal inhabited pockets of Madhya Pradesh State. These taxa are used for curing various ailments among the different ethnic societies of Madhya Pradesh. The information has been gathered by field survey and also from available literature. For the first time here is a detailed explaination of 266 Ethnomedicinal plants of Madhya Pradesh with vernacular names, distribution, Botanical description, flowering & fruiting, medicinal parts, chemical constituents, Ethnomedicinal/Folk uses and Ayurvedic Medicinal uses as described in Ancient Ayurvedic Literature. The need for the present work has been felt by the author to provide basic information to pharmaceutical industries and various other organizations working on the traditional system of medicines. The information of all potential medicinal plants based on folk claims and data recorded from literature have been incorporated so that the natural resources may be utilized as an alternative source of drugs for the welfare of mankind without affecting the natural ecosystem. This book well helps in generating an interest in ethnomedicinal plants of Madhya Pradesh.

I hope that this compilation of most commonly used ethnomedicinal plants will be of use to Ethnobotanists, Ayurvedic practitioners, students and researchers as well as to medical and scientific communities worked on the medicinal and ethnomedicinal plants of Madhya Pradesh.

Dinesh Jadhav

Contents

Introduction

Man has depended on plants from time immemorial; plants have been a rich source for therapeutics (Ambasta 1986; Anonymous 1948-1976; Lindley 1981; Verma and Tewari 2016.). Medicinal plants belong to the earliest known health care products that have been used by the mankind. Most of the drug yielding plants are found in the tropics growing in wild condition and are mainly used by herb doctors and Ayurvedic vaidyas, who refer to them as *jari-butis* (Gogte and Vaidya 2000; Handa and Kapoor 1999; Khory 1981; Mishra and Vaisya 2004). While humans suffered in olden times from innumerable maladies and diseases, they experimented with plant cures. The primitive people are well acquainted with the properties and uses of plants of their surroundings. They have inherited rich traditional knowledge (TK) of surrounding plants. Such knowledge of economic and other properties of surrounding plants acquired by the tribal community through experience of ages has been passed on the word of mouth from generation to generation as a part of their cultural heritage. Many prescriptions are based on experimentation and observations. In the modern age with the fast emergence of western modern medicine and synthetic drugs, the importance of plants and herbs started declining as more and more attention was paid to the development of synthetic drugs. However, with these synthetic drug came the problems of side effects and other clinical complications; the reason in the increasing awareness about the limitations of the synthetic drugs. Because of natural herbal drugs being safe and effective; now herbal medicines and natural products are in big demand all over the World. Over three-quarters of the World population rely on the use of traditional medicines for their primary health care needs. The medicinal plants are not only major components of the many formulations used in indigenous systems of medicine but also of a large number of drugs in Allopathy. In India, with one of the oldest ethnobotanical tradition in the World, medicinal plants are the backbone of all major systems of medicine. One of the earliest references to the Medicinal properties of plants is in the *Rigveda* (3500 - 1800 BC). *Ayurveda*, the ancient Indian system of medicine based on that medicinal property of plants (Pandey, 1969; Sharma, 2003). Ayurvedic text manifests that an incredible 1600 of the 2000 old Ayurvedic formulations are plant based. About two thousand plants are mentioned in the Ayurvedic system of medicine (Chopra *et al.,* 1956; Gupta and Tandon, 2004; Joshi, 2007; Kirtikar and Basu, 2004; Paranjpe, 2005; Warrier *et al.,* 1994). There are many more useful medicinal plants has been described under Ayurvedic medicinal system by several authors at that time i.e. '*Charakh*' and '*Susruta*' etc (Printya, 1963; Sharma and Bhagvan dash, 1976). After that there are many more books have been written under heading medicinal plants of India and Madhya Pradesh, but they could not fulfil all the requirements of research scholar and readers who worked/interested in the field of Ethnomedicinal Plants of Madhya Pradesh. Presently, there are a number of ethnobotanical studies in different tribal inhabited localities of Madhya Pradesh are being carried out actively. Ethnobotanical work done in Madhya Pradesh in last 7 decades has led to the publication of inventories and documentation of plants and their products used by the aboriginals for various purposes. Madhya Pradesh state is rich not only in floristic diversity but also in tribal or ethnic diversity. A large number of ethnobotanical papers on the region is scattered in various journals, magazines, books, proceedings, etc. The present book deals the ethnomedicinal wealth of Madhya Pradesh state. The ethnobotanical information has already been recorded to some extent by the earlier workers. These workers have contributed to our knowledge about various ethnobotanical and ethnomedicinal data on numerous plants. The present book deals with the 266 species of probable Ethnomedicinal potential from tribal inhabited pockets of Madhya Pradesh State. These taxa are used for curing various ailments among the different ethnic societies of Madhya Pradesh. The information has been gathered by field survey and also from available literature.

Study Area

In India, Madhya Pradesh is known to harbour a rich wealth of Medicinal Plants. The State lies in the central region of the Country between latitudes 21^0 6' – 26^0 30' N and longitudes 74^0 9' – 81^0 48' E covers an area of 3,08,245 sq. km. Uttar Pradesh bound it in the North, Chhattisgarh in the East, Maharashtra in the South and Rajasthan and Gujarat in the West. It comprises 45 districts, *viz.*, Balaghat, Barwani, Betul, Bhind, Bhopal, Chhatarpur, Chhindwara, Damoh, Datia, Dewas, Dhar, Dindori, East Nimar (Khandwa), Guna, Gwalior, Harda, Hoshangabad, Indore, Jabalpur, Jhabua, Katni, Mandala, Mandsaur, Morena, Narsinhpur, Neemuch, Omaria, Panna, Raisen, Rajgarh, Ratlam, Rewa, Sagar, Satna, Sehore, Seoni, Shahdol, Shajapur, Shivpuri, Sheopur, Sidhi, Tikamgarh, Ujjain, Vidisha, West Nimar (Khargone) (Fig. 1.). With respect to forest cover, it is the first largest state in India. The forests that account for 30.9% of the total geographical area cover about 95,211 sq km area. The forests are dominated by Teak (*Tectona grandis*) and Sal (*Shorea robusta*). The major rivers are Narmada, Chambal, Kalisindh, Betwa, Son, Venganga, Mahi, Tapti, Ken and Pench. The climate of the state is generally sub-humid with an annual rainfall ranging from 75-125 cm. The minimum and maximum temperatures range between 2^0 C and 45 ^{0}C in the months of January and May, respectively. According to 2001 census, the total population of the state is about 6,03,48,023, out of which 1,22,33,474 (20.27%) from 41 tribal communities, which are divided into more than 59 ethnic groups. The main tribes and their sub-tribes of the state are Agaria, Baiga (Binjhwar, Narotia, Bharotia, Nahar, Re-bhena, Kad-bhena), Basor, Bharia (Bhumia, Bhuihar, Pando), Bhil (Bhilala, Berela, Patlia), Gond (Pardhan, Agaria, Ojha, Nagarchi, Solhas), Halba (Halbi), Kanjar, Khairwar, Kol (Rhoeo, Rothel), Kondar, Korku (Nahala, Bodoya), Pao (Pabra), Madia (Abhujmadia, Dandami Madia, Metakoitur), Mawasi, Mobasi, Oroan, Sahariya, Sor. The economy of the state is primarily agriculture based. The state is famous for Soya bean cultivation and is known as the 'Soya bean state'. Nearly 75% of the population lives in villages. The life of villagers is wholly or partially dependent upon forest resources. They utilize a wide variety of plants for their basic needs, such as food, fibre, fodder, wood, medicine, gum, tannin, resin, dye and shelter.

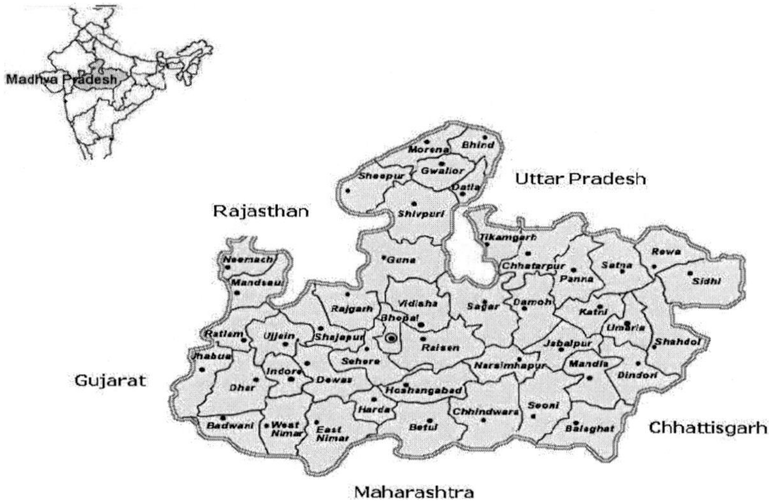

Fig. 1. Map of Madhya Pradesh

Ethnomedicinal Plants of Madhya Pradesh

1. *Abelmoschus esculentus* (L.) Moench. (Malvaceae)

Syn.: *Hibiscus esculentus* L.

Vern.: Bhindi.

Distribution: Commonly cultivated throughout the State.

Botany: Hispidly hairy herb, with 3 to 7-lobed leaves and yellow flowers with purple centre. Fruits cylendric, 5-angled, beaked. Flowering & Fruiting: April-September.

Medicinal Parts: Root.

Chemical Constituents: Fruits contain 5-hydroxytryptamin, oxalates, iodine, flourine, Calcium, phosphorus, Magnesium, vitamin-C, fats, carbohydrates, fibres, Amino-acids, Polyphenols.

Folk Use: Aphrodisiac, Spermatorrhoea

Use in literature: Fruits- Abdominal disorders, anaemia, diarrhoea, dysuria, gonorrhoea, Pruritus, spermatorrhoea.

Seeds- Gonorrhoea.

2. *Abelmoschus moschatus* (L.) Medic. (Malvaceae)

Syn.: *Hibiscus abelmoschus* L.

Vern.: Kasturi Bhindi, Mushk dana.

Distribution: In mixed forests and along cultivated fields. Mandla.

Botany: Strigose undershrubs, with ovate-cordate leaves. Flowers bright yellow with dark purple centre. Capsules acuminate, villous. Seeds reniform. Flowering & Fruiting: September – October.

Medicinal Parts: Seeds.

Chemical constituents: Seeds contains Farnesol, ambrettolide, sterols, terpenes and aliphatic compounds.

Seed oil contains 12, 13 – epoxyoleic acid, malvalic acid, sterculic acid & phospholipids.

Folk Use: Hysteria, Itches

Use in literature: Seeds – Dyspepsia, flatulence, gonorrhoea, hysteria, intestinal complaints, itching, leucoderma, nervous debility, snakebite, stomatitis, urinary discharges, vomiting.

3. *Abrus precatorius* L. (Papilionaceae)

Syn.: *Glycine abrus* L.

Vern.: Ratti.

Distribution: On roadside trees and shrubs. Balaghat, Bhopal, Damoh, Hoshangabad, Indore, Jabalpur, Mandla, Panna, Raisen, Ratlam, Rewa, Sagar, Satna, Seoni, Shahdol, Shivpuri, Sidhi, W. Nimar.

Botany: Twining shrubs, with 10-20 pairs of leaflets and pink or white flowers having 9 stamens. Pods 3-5 seeded. Flowering & Fruiting: August-February.

Medicinal Parts: Leaves, Roots, Seeds.

Chemical constituents: Root contains Stigmasterol, Glycine, Glutamic acid, Aspartic acid, Tyrosin, Quercetin, Luteplin, Kaempferol, Taxalbumin; Alkaloid-abrin; Glucoside-abralin; Anthocyanin-abranin.

Seeds contain Lupeol acetate, Sitosterol, Sucrose, Gallic acid, Orietin, Isoorientin, Abrussic acid, Haemagglutinin.

Leaves contain Precol, Abrol, Abrasine, Precasine.

Folk Use: Cold, Cough, Hoarseness, Intestinal worms, Prevent conception, Rheumatism, Urinary diseases

Use in literature: Root – Asthma, biliousness, colic, fever, gonorrhoea, Jaundice, stomatitis, tuberculous glands.

Leaves – Asthma, cold, colic, cough, fever, gonorrhoea, headache, hoarseness, itching, jaundice, leucoderma, skin diseases, stomatitis, swelling, tuberculous glands.

Seeds – Diarrhoea, dysentery, leprosy, nervous disorders, paralysis, sciatica, ulcer.

4. *Abutilon indicum* (L.) Sweet (Malvaceae)

Syn.: *Abutilon asiaticum* (L.) Sweet.; *Sida guineensis* Schum.

Vern.: Kanghi.

Distribution: In Wastelands, Stream sides and Hill slopes. Balaghat, Bhopal, Damoh, Indore, Panna, Satna, Shahdol, Sidhi.

Botany: Undershrubs, with ovate – suborbicular leaves and axillary, solitary flowers. Fruits with 15-25 mericarps.

Flowering & Fruiting: September – January.

Medicinal Parts: Root, Leaves.

Chemical constituents: Plant contains Gossypetin, Glucosides, Cyanidin, Rutinosides, essential oil.

Root contains Fatty acids, Aspargin, Rafinose.

Stem & Leaves contain Alkanol, Beta–Sitosterol, Vanillic acid, Caffeic acid, Fumaric acid, Fructose, Glucose, Galactose, Leucin, Histidine, Threonine, Serine, Glutamic acid and Aspartic acid.

Folk Use: Boils, Leucorrhoea

Use in literature: Root – Eye diseases, fever, leprosy, leucoderma, Piles, stone in bladder, strangury, uterine hemorrhagic discharges.

Root bark – Strangury, urinary complaints.

Leaves – Boils, bronchitis, diarrhoea, fever, gonorrhoea, gums, inflammation, lumbago, piles, toothache, ulcers, vaginal infections, wounds.

Seeds – Bronchitis, chronic chest trouble, cough, cystitis, gleet, gonorrhoea, piles.

5. *Acacia arabica* auct. (Mimosaceae)

Syn.: *A. nilotica* (L.) Willd. ex Delile ssp. *indica* (Benth.) Brenan.

Vern.: Babool.

Distribution: In dry deciduous forests and roadsides. Balaghat, Bhind, Bhopal, Chhatarpur, Damoh, Gwalior, Hosahangabad, Indore, Mandla, Panna, Raisen, Sagar, Satna, Seoni, Shivpuri, Sidhi.

Botany: Trees, with long, white stipular spines. Pinnae 2-11 pairs and leaflets 7-25 pairs. Heads bright yellow, axillary, pedunculate, pods moniliform.

Flowering & Fruiting: July – January.

Medicinal Parts: Leaves, Stem bark.

Chemical constituents: Bark contains Beta-amyrin, Gallic acid, tannins, catechin, quercetin, leucocyanidin.

Fruit contains Gallic Acid, Catechin, Chlorogenic acid.

Gum contains Galactose, Arabic Acid, Calcium, Magnesium.

Seeds contains Ascorbic acid, Niacin, Thiamine, Amino acids.

Folk Use: Cough, Diabetes, Diarrhoea, Dysentery, Menstrual bleeding, Piles

Use in literature: Gum – Biliousness, bone fractures, diabetes, diarrhoea, dysentery, leprosy, sore throat, urinary discharges.

Stem bark – Biliousness, bronchitis, burning sensation, cough, diarrhoea, dysentery, leucoderma, piles, urinary discharges.

Fruit – Biliousness.

Leaves – bone fractures, bronchitis, eye diseases, gonorrhoea, piles.

6. *Acacia catechu* Willd. (Mimosaceae)

Syn.: *Mimosa catechu* L. f.; *M. catechuoides* Roxb.

Vern.: Khair.

Distribution: In dry deciduous forests. Balaghat, Bhopal, Chhindwada, E. Nimarh, Gwalior, Hosahangabad, Indore, Jabalpur, Mandla, Panna, Raisen, Sagar, Satna, Shivpuri, Sidhi.

Botany: Trees; all part pubescent; prickles hooked. Leaves 2-pinnate, with glands on the petiole and between the pinnae; leaflets 10-30 pairs. Spikes pale yellow. Pods flat. Flowering & Fruiting: May – September.

Medicinal Parts: Stem bark, Root.

Chemical constituents: Inner wood contains Catechin & Catechutannic acid (Catechutannic acid contain about 50% Tannin).

Folk Use: Cough, Dysentery, Oral ulcer, Rheumatism

Use in literature: Stem bark – Anaemia, boils, bronchitis, cough, diarrhoea, diseases of the tooth, elephantiasis, erysipelas, heaviness, indigestion, inflammation, itching, leprosy, leucoderma, psoriasis, sore throat, skin diseases, ulcers, urinary discharges, worms.

Resinous extract – Cough, diarrhoea, leprosy, leucoderma, leucorrhoea, oedema, piles, throat diseases, toothache, ulcer, urinary diseases, vaginal discharges.

7. *Acacia leucophloea* (Roxb.) Willd. (Mimosaceae)

Syn.: *A. alba* Willd; *Mimosa leucophloea* Roxb.

Vern.: Safed babool.

Distribution: In wastelands and roadsides. Balaghat, Bhopal, Bhind, Dhar, Gwalior, Hosahangabad, Indore, Mandla, Morena, Panna, Raisen, Ratlam, Sagar, Satna, Seoni, Shivpuri, Sidhi, Tikamgarh.

Botany: Trees, with stipular-spines in pairs. Pinnae 3-15 pairs with concave glands in between and 5-30 pairs of leaflets. Heads pale-yellow, in terminal panicles. Pods flat, linear. Flowering & Fruiting: May-March.

Medicinal Parts: Root, StemBark.

Chemical constituents: Stem Bark contain n-hexacosanol, β-amyrin, β-sitosterol, tannin, isookannin, cyanin, leuoxol.

Heartwood contain n-hexacosanol, β-amyrin.

Folk Use: Diarrhoea, Fever

Use in literature: Bark – Bronchitis, cough, diarrhoea, dysentery, erysipelas, fever, inflammation, leprosy, leucoderma, pruritus, skin diseases, ulcers, vomiting, wounds.

8. *Acalypha indica* L. (Euphorbiaceae)

Vern.: Kuppi.

Distribution: Common as weed in gardens, fields, old buildings and vacant plots near villages. Chhatarpur, Dhar, Indore.

Botany: Erect herbs, with ovate or ovate – rhomboid leaves. Flowers greenish, in androgynous spikes; bracts concealing the capsules, Shortly dentate, capsules hispid. Flowering & Fruiting: July-November.

Medicinal Parts: Whole plant.

Chemical constituents: Plant contains Kaempferol, Acalyphamide, sterols, cyanogenic glyceride.

Folk Use: Asthma, Bronchities, Pneumonia

Use in literature: Whole Plant – Asthma, arthritis, bronchitis, burns, earache, pneumonia, ringworm, scabies, skin diseases, snake-bite, toothache.

9. *Achyranthes aspera* L. (Amaranthaceae)

Vern.: Apamarg, Latjira.

Distribution: Common in wastelands. Balaghat, Bhopal, Chhatarpur, Damoh, Jabalpur, Narsimhapur, Panna, Rewa, Satna, Seoni, Sidhi, Tikamgarh.

Botany: Erect hairy herbs, with oval–round pubescent- villous leaves. Flowers rather plump in appearance, deflexed, spinescent, in lax spikes.

Flowering & Fruiting: August- February.

Medicinal Parts: Whole plant, Leaves, Roots, Seeds.

Chemical constituents: Seed contains Saponin A & B, Ecdy steron, oligosaccharide.

Root contains Oleonilic acid, maslinic acid.

Unripe fruit contains Saponin C & D.

Plant contains Nitrogenous compound- Achranthine & alkaloids.

Folk Use: Asthma, Dental pain, Snake bite, Scorpion sting, Stone trouble, Fever.

Use in literature: Root- Abdominal pain, blood diseases, cancer, colic, deafness, disease of the tooth, heart diseases, itching, leucoderma, liver disorders, stone in bladder, tumor, vomiting, wound.

Leaves – Gonorrhoea, leprosy.

Seeds – Cold, colic, cough, hydrophobia, leprosy, scabies, toothache.

10. *Acorus calamus* L. (Araceae)

Vern.: Bach

Distribution: Rare. In marshy places.

Botany: Small aquatic or marshy herb, with tuberous fleshy, creeping aromatic cylindrical rhizome; leaves linear, strap shaped.

Flowering & Fruiting: July-September.

Medicinal Parts: Rhizome, Root.

Chemical constituents: Rhizome contains Essential oil, Glucoside-Acorin.

Leaves contain Oxalic acid, Calcium, Asarone, Chlorpromazine.

Folk Use: Snake bite, Stomachache

Use in literature: Rhizome – Amenorrhoea, bronchitis, calculi, colic, cough, depression, dysentery, dysmenorrhoea, dyspepsia, epilepsy, fever, flatulence, gout, helminthiasis, hoarseness, inflammations, otalgia, skin diseases, strangury, tumours.

11. *Adhatoda zeylanica Medic.* (Acanthaceae)

Syn.: *A. vasica* Nees.; *Justicia adhatoda* L.

Vern.: Adusa.

Distribution: Common in fields and wastelands. Chhatarpur, Damoh, Hosahangabad, Indore, Rewa, Satna, Seoni.

Botany: Shrubs, with elliptic leaves. Flowers white or creamish- white in elongate spikes; corolla – tube mottled. Capsules 4 – seeded. Flowering & Fruiting: December-March.

Medicinal Parts: Leaves.

Chemical constituents: Leaves contains A bitter vasicine, Adhatodic acid, volatile oil, vasa, Resin, gum, sugar & yellow pigment.

Plant contains Alkaloids (Vasicoline, Adhatodine, Vasicolinine, Anisolin), Vasicine & Vasicinone.

Folk Use: Asthma, Bronchitis, Cough, Rheumatism, Tuberculosis

Use in literature: Asthma, blood impurities, chronic bronchitis, cold, cough, diseases of the mouth, fever, gonorrhoea, haemorrhagic diseases, heart troubles, jaundice, leprosy, ophthalmia, respiratory disorders, rheumatism, skin diseases, tumors, urinary diseases, whooping cough.

12. *Aegle marmelos* (L.) Corr. ex Roxb. (Rutaceae)

Vern.: Bel, Bilvapatra.

Distribution: Balaghat, Damoh, Dhar, Hosahangabad, Panna, Seoni, Tikamgarh.

Botany: Deciduous trees, armed with spines. Leaves 3- foliolate and flowers creamy – white in axillary panicles. Fruits globose with stony rind and mucilaginous pulp. Flowering & Fruiting: March – April.

Medicinal Parts: Leaves, fruits.

Chemical constituents: Fruits contains Gum, pectins, reducing sugars, sugars, oil, and tannin.

Leaves & Root contains Reducing sugars, Tannins, Iron, Calcium, Magnesium, and Potassium.

Folk Use: Abdominal disorders, Asthma, Dysentery, Vomiting.

Use in literature: Ripe fruit – Diarrhoea, biliousness, dysentery, dyspepsia.

Root – Abdominal pain, colic, fever, dyspepsia, dysuria, nervous disorders, oedema, rheumatism, urinary trouble, vomiting.

Leaves – Deafness, inflammation, ophthalmia.

13. *Aerva lanata* (L.) Juss. ex Schultes (Amaranthaceae)

Syn.: *Achyrantuhus lantana* L.; *Celosia lanata* L.

Vern.: Gorakhganja.

Distribution: Common as weed in wastelands, along river banks and roadsides. Balaghat, Betul, Chhatarpur, Damoh, Dhar, E. Nimar, Hosahangabad, Indore, Mandla, Panna, Ratlam, Rewa, Satna, Seoni, Sidhi, Tikamgarh, W. Nimar..

Botany: Perennial herbs, with suborbicular to lanceolate leaves. Flowers bisexual, in axillary spikes passing into long leafy inflorescence. Fruits rotund, compressed. Flowering & Fruiting: July-April.

Medicinal Parts: Dried Flower.

Chemical constituents: α-Amyrin, campesterol, β-sitosterol, palmitic acid, betuline, syringic acid, vanllic acid, feruloyltyramine, aervine, methylervine, aervoside, aervolanine.

Folk Use: Kidney stone.

Use in literature: Plant – Boils, Cough, Strangury.

14. *Ageratum conyzoides* L. (Asteraceae)

Vern.: Osdi, Sadoradi.

Distribution: Common weed of moist places along the irrigation channels and strems. Balaghat, Hoshangabad, Sidhi.

Botany: An annual hairy herb; leaves ovate – cordate, serrate; heads white in terminal corymbs. Flowering & Fruiting: Round the year.

Medicinal Parts: Leaves, Root, Whole plant.

Chemical constituents: Essential oil, Saponins, Flavonoids, alkaloids, amino acids, sugars, Vitamin – A & B.

Folk Use: Cuts, Headache, Leucoderma

Use in literature: Leaf – Eye diseases, Leprosy, tetanus, wound.

Root – Eye diseases.

15. *Ailanthus excelsa* Roxb. (Simaroubaceae)

Vern.: Maharukh.

Distribution: Chhatarpur, Hosahangabad, Indore, Jabalpur, Seoni, Shivpuri, Sidhi.

Botany: Large trees, with pinnate leaves crowned at the end of branches. Flowers yellow, in terminal and axillary panicles. Fruit a samara, spindle shaped, 1-seeded. Flowering & Fruiting: December-April.

Medicinal Parts: Leaves, Stem bark.

Chemical constituents: Bark contains Glaucarubin, Glauca rubinone, Excelsin, Glaucarubol, Ailanthion, Ailantic acid, Malantahin, Tricontane, Hexatricontane.

Leaves contain Ailantic acid, Beta – sitosterol (vitexin).

Folk Use: Asthma, Bronchitis, Debility, Fever, Typhoid

Use in literature: Stem bark – Asthma, bronchitis, chronic fever, diarrhoea, dysentery, dyspepsia, earache, leprosy, piles, skin diseases, vomiting, worm infestation.

16. *Alangium salvifolium* (L.f.) Wang. (Alangiaceae)

Syn.: *A. lamarckii* Thw.; *Grewia salvifolium* (L. f.) Suppl.

Vern.: Ankol.

Distribution: Damoh, Mandla.

Botany: A small tree with spinescent branches and grey bark. Leaves simple, alternate, membranous, varying in size and shape. Flowers in axillary clusters, small, white, and fragrant. Fruits berry, globular, crowned with persistent calyx-limb, purplish-red to black. Flowering & Fruiting: February– May.

Medicinal Parts: Leaves.

Chemical constituents: Flower contain Deoxytubulosine alkaloid.

Fruits contain Cephaeline, deoxytubulosine, alangside, sterol, N-methylcephaeline.

Seed containAlamarckine, emetin, cephaeline, isocephaeline & other alkaloids.

Leaves contain Alkaloids, sterols & terpenoids.

Stem bark contain Tubulosine, cephaeline, psychotrine alkaloids.

Folk Use: Piles, Rheumatism, Scorpion sting

Use in literature: Root bark – Colic, biliousness, fever, skin diseases.

Leaves- Rheumatic pain.

Fruits – Haemorrhages.

Seed – Boils, Haemorrhages.

17. *Albizia lebbeck* (L.) Willd. (Mimosaceae)

Syn.: *Mimosa lebbeck* L.; *Acacia speciosa* Willd.

Vern.: Sirus.

Distribution: In mixed forests and roadsides. Bhopal, Damoh, Gwalior, E. Nimar, Hosahangabad, Indore, Jabalpur, Panna, Raisen, Sagar, Shivpuri.

Botany: Deciduous trees, with 1-4 pairs of pinnae and 4-10 pairs of leaflets. Flowers pale-green, in umbellate heads. Pods flat, straw-coloured.

Flowering & Fruiting: April-September.

Medicinal Parts: Seed.

Chemical constituents: Bark contains Tannins, saponin, Echinocytic acid, and β- sitosterol.

Pods contain Saponins, Echinocytic acid, Olionilic acid, Albigenine & Albigenic acid, lebbekanin – C, Glucose & Rhamnose.

Seed contains Triterpenic saponin.

Folk Use: Piles, Skin diseases

Use in literature: Stem bark – Asthma, blood disorders, bronchitis, conjunctivitis, cough, diarrhoea, eczema, erysipelas, helmintic inflammation, itching, leprosy, leucoderma, malaria, migraine, Oedema, paralysis, piles, Rhinitis, sinusitis, skin diseases, snake bite, ulcer, urticaria, worm Infestation.

Root bark – Good for gums.

Leaves – Nightblindness, Ophthalmia.

Seed – Gonorrhoea.

18. *Allium cepa* L. (Liliaceae)

Vern.: Piyaz.

Distribution: Cultivated throughout the State.

Botany: An annual herb, with bulbous stem, fistular, linear leaves and white flowers in umbels.

Flowering & Fruiting: December-March.

Medicinal Parts: Bulb.

Chemical constituents: Bulb contains Glutamyl, Arginin, Cystein, Quercetin, Kaempferol, Methylcystein, Sulphoxide, Propylecystein, Saponins.

Folk Use: Cholera, Snake bite

Use in literature: Anti-tumour, bronchitis, dysentery, gum swelling, Jaundice, night blindness, piles.

19. *Allium sativum* L. (Liliaceae)

Vern.: Lasun.

Distribution: Cultivated throughout the State.

Botany: Bulbous herbs, each bulb with several fleshy bulblets. Leaves linear. Flowers white, in umbels.

Flowering & Fruiting: December-March.

Medicinal Parts: Bulb.

Chemical constituents: Bulb contains A volatile oil which contains Allyl disulphide, Allyl-propyl disulphide and Poly sulphide; Allicin (antibacterial): Allicetion-I and Allicetion-II (Antibiotics).

Folk Use: Asthma, Ringworm

Use in literature: Asthma, bronchitis, chronic cough, ear trouble, epilepsy, flatulence, malaria fever, skin diseases, tuberculosis, ulcer.

20. *Aloe vera* L. (Liliaceae)

Syn.: *A. barbadensis* Mill.

Vern.: Gwarpatha.

Distribution: Cultivated throughout the State, sometimes wild in drier localities.

Botany: Perennial herbs, with fleshy mucilaginous leaves in rosette having marginal spines. Flowers yellow, born in racemes on long scapes.

Flowering & Fruiting: November-March.

Medicinal Parts: Pulp of leaves.

Chemical constituents: Leaves contain Carbohydrates, Tannins, Proteins, Chromones (Abesin & Aloesone), Malic acid, Citric acid, Tartaric acid.

Jelly from leaves contain Acetylated glucomannans, Iron, Calcium, Potassium & Magnesium.

Folk Use: Headache, Rheumatism

Use in literature: Leaf pulp – Cold, colic, constipation, cough, fever, menstrual disorders, piles, rectal fissures, rheumatism.

21. *Alstonia scholaris* R. Br. (Apocynaceae)

Syn.: *A. cuneata* Wall.

Vern.: Chatium, Saptparni.

Distribution: Planted. Indore.

Botany: A large tree with whorled branches and leaves with bitter milky juice, white flowers.

Flowering & Fruiting: December-June.

Medicinal Parts: Stem Bark.

Chemical constituents: Leaves contain Picralinol, Akuammigine, Tubotaiwine, Akuammicine.

Flowers contain Picrinine, Strictamine, Tetrahydro alstonic, Hexacosane, Lupeol, Beta-Amyrin, Palmitic acid, Urolic acid.

Stem bark contain Echitamine, Venoterpine-Glucoside.

Folk Use: Diarrhoea, Dysentery

Use in literature: Dropsy, dysentery, gastro-intestinal troubles, malaria, ulcers.

22. *Alternanthera sessilis* (L.) R. Br. ex. DC. (Amaranthaceae)

Syn.: *A. triandra* Lam.; *A. denticulata* R. Br.; *A. nodiflora* R. Br.

Vern.: Guroo.

Distribution: Common in aquatic and semi-aquatic situations. Balaghat, Betul, Chhatarpur, Damoh, E. Nimar, Dhar, Guna, Gwalior, Hosahangabad, Indore, Jabalpur, Mandla, Panna, Rewa, Sagar, Satna, Seoni, Shivpuri, Sidhi, Tikamgarh.

Botany: A prostrate or spreading, polymorphic herbs; stem grooved, greenish-purple, with white hairy appendages, much branched, often rooting at the nodes; leaves glabrous, elliptic, linear-oblong, cuneate at the base, acute; flowers in axillary, small, white or pink-tinged, spicate-heads; seeds minute. Flowering & Fruiting: Throughout the year.

Medicinal Parts: Whole plant.

Plant contains Iron, protein, hydrocarbons & sterols.

Folk Use: Gynaecological disorders.

Use in literature: Dried plant – Blood disorders, leprosy.

Root – Wound.

23. *Amaranthus spinosus* L. (Amaranthaceae)

Vern.: Kantili chauli.

Distribution: Common in wastelands and disturbed area along roadsides. Balaghat, Chhatarpur, Damoh, Indore, Jabalpur, Mandla, Panna, Rewa, Satna, Shahdol, Sidhi, Tikamgarh, W. Nimar.

Botany: Monoecious herb, with ovate-rhomboid or elliptic leaves having axillary spines. Flowers in axillary clusters, passing to spikes. Fruits ovoid. Flowering & Fruiting: Throughout the year.

Medicinal Parts: Root.

Chemical constituents: Plant contains Carbohydrates, Proteins, Minerals, Iron, Vitamin – A and Calcium (Leaves).

Folk Use: Cold, Cough

Use in literature: Biliousness, blood diseases, burning sensation, bronchitis, hallucination, leprosy, leucorrhoea, piles.

24. *Amaranthus tricolor* L. (Amaranthaceae)

Syn.: *A. tristis* L.; *A. gangeticus* L.; *A. melancholius* L.; *A. polygamus* L.

Distribution: Common as weed in wastelands & Cultivated fields, also cultivated. Balaghat, Chhatarpur, Damoh, Gwalior, Mandla, Satna, Shahdol, Sidhi, W. Nimar.

Botany: Ascending herbs; Stems angular; flowers densely Clustered in interrupted spikes. Flowering & Fruiting: August-October.

Medicinal parts: Seed.

Chemical constituents:

Leaves – Amino acids, Calcium, Magnesium, Mangnese, Phosphorus, Iron, Amaranthine, Cholesterol, Campesterol, Stigmasterol, Fucosterol, Glucose, Fructose, Isoamaranthine.

Folk Use: Rheumatism

Use in literature: Dysentery, Haemoptysis.

25. *Ammania baccifera* L. (Lythraceae)

Vern.: Dadamari

Syn.: *A. salicifolia* Hiern.; *A. vesicatoria* Roxb.

Distribution: Balaghat, Damoh, Gwalior, Hosahangabad, Indore, Jabalpur, Mandla, Morena, Narsimhapur, Rewa, Sagar, Satna, Seoni, Sidhi.

Botany: Erect or ascending herbs, with oblong or elliptic leaves and sessile flowers lacking petals and style. Capsules globose, reddish.

Flowering & Fruiting: November-April.

Medicinal Parts: Leaves.

Chemical constituents: Hentriaconite, Dotriacontanol, Betulinic acid, Lupeol, Ellagic acid, Quercetin, Lawsone.

Folk Use: Rheumatism

Use in literature: Plant – Burning sensation, colic, dyspepsia, fever, flatulence, rheumatism, seminal weakness, strangury.

26. *Amorphophallus campanulatus* (Roxb.) Blume ex Decne (Araceae)

Vern.: Jangali suran.

Distribution: In shady places. Indore.

Botany: A perennial herb. Tubers depressed-globose, bulbiferous, dark brown. Leaves very large, arising after the flowers, long with pale blotches, stout; leaflets obovate; flowers in long spadix.

Flowering & Fruiting: July-October.

Medicinal Parts: Corm.

Chemical constituents: Corm contains Proteins, fats, Carbohydrate, Minerals, Calcium Oxalate, Phosphorous, Iron, vitamin A & B.

Folk Use: Piles, Rheumatism

Use in literature: Corm – Asthma, colic, cough, dysentery flatulence, gastric trouble, piles, rheumatism, vomiting, worms.

27. *Ampelocissus latifolia* (Roxb.) Planch. (Vitaceae)

Syn.: *Vitis latifolia* Roxb.

Vern.: Panibel.

Distribution: Balaghat, Damoh, Hosahangabad, Mandla, Rewa, Satna, Seoni, Shivpuri.

Botany: Large climbers, with hollow, striate branches. Leaves orbicular-cordate, lobed, serrate. Flowers reddish-brown, in pyramidal thyrsoid cymes.berries globose, black, 2-seeded.

Flowering & Fruiting: Agust-November.

Medicinal Parts: Leaves, Root.

Chemical Constituents: Root contains Saponins

Folk Use: Dental trouble, Dysentery, Rheumatism

Use in literature: Root – Chronic, Dysentery, Wounds.

Leaf – Dental problem, Indolent ulcers, Wounds.

28. *Andrographis paniculata* (Burm. f.) Wall. ex Nees (Acanthaceae)

Syn.: *A. subspathulata* Clarke; *Justicia Paniculata* Burm.

Vern.: Kalmegh.

Distribution: Common in wastelands. Balaghat, Bhopal, Chhatarpur, Damoh, Hosahangabad, Narsimhapur, Sidhi.

Botany: Erect, glabrous, annual. Branches 4-angled. Leaves slightly undulate; base tapering. Flowers small, solitary, whitish, spotted with rose-purple. Corolla 2-lipped. Capsules linear-oblong.

Flowering & Fruiting: September-April.

Medicinal Parts: Whole plant.

Chemical constituents: Plant contains Kalmeghin, Andrographolid, Tannic acid, Sodium and Potassium.

Folk Use: Snake bite.

Use in literature: Anorexia, blood purifier, hepatomegally, malaria, oedema, skin diseases.

29. *Anethum graveolens* L. (Apiaceae)

Syn.: *Peucedanum graveolens* (L.) Hiren.; *P. sowa* Roxb.; *Anethum sowa* Roxb. ex Flem.

Vern.: Sowa.

Distribution: Chhatarpur.

Botany: A glabrous aromatic annual herb; leaves pinnately compound; flowers yellow, in compound umbels.

Flowering & Fruiting: January-March.

Medicinal Parts: Fruits, Seeds.

Chemical constituents: Fruits contain Vicenin, Phellandrene, Dillapiol, Carvone, Dihydro carvone, D-limonene, A new xanthone glycoside-dillanoside.

Seed oil contain Essential oil, Tripetroselinin, Petroselinicdiolein, Dipetroselinicolein.

Folk Use: Menorrhoea, Lactation

30. *Anisomeles indica* (L.) Kuntze. (Lamiaceae)

Syn.: *A. ovata* R. Br.

Distribution: As forest undergrowth, on hill slopes and roadsides. Balaghat, Chhindwara, Damoh, Gwalior, Hosahangabad, Indore, Mandla, Panna, Rewa, Sagar, Seoni, Sidhi.

Botany: Suffruticose herbs, with ovate, acute or obtuse, crenate-serrate, softe, softly pubescent leaves. Flowers bluish-purple. Nutlets broadly ovoid, with rounded ends, polished. Flowering & Fruiting: August-March.

Medicinal Parts: Leaves.

Chemical Constituents: The plant contains Essential oil.

Folk Use: Peptic ulcer, Rickets

Use in literature: Essential oil from plant – Uterine affections.

31. *Annona squamosa* L. (Annonaceae)

Vern.: Seetaphaal.

Distribution: Cultivated in gardens for its edible fruits as well as an escape along forest margins. dry deciduous forests and roadsides. Balaghat, Damoh, Dhar, Hosahangabad, Indore, Mandla, Rewa, Seoni, Tikamgarh.

Botany: Evergreen shrubs or small trees with oblong-lanceolate leaves and yellowish green flowers. Fruits globose or ovoid with projecting areoles.

Flowering & Fruiting: July – November.

Medicinal Parts: Seeds.

Chemical constituents: Leaves contain Anonaine, Roemerine, Corydine, Narcorydine, Norlaureline, Isocorydine, Noricocorydine, Glucine, Friedeline, Alkaloids, Essential oils, Volatile oil, Carvone, Michelabine, Liriodedine, Diazepine, Squamolone, Beta–Caryophylline, β-sitosterol, Camphor, Barmeol.

Folk Use: Prevent conception

Use in literature: Bark **–** Diarrhoea.

Leaves – Boils, swelling, ulcers.

Fruits- Diarrhoea, dysentery, dyspepsia, vertigo, vomiting.

32. *Anogeissus latifolia* (Roxb. ex DC.) Wall. ex Guill. & Perr. (Combretaceae)

Vern.: Dhawra.

Distribution: In dry deciduous forests. Balaghat, Bhopal, Damoh, E. Nimar, Guna, Hosahangabad, Indore, Jabalpur, Mandla, Narsimhapur, Panna, Raisen, Rewa, Sagar, Satna, Seoni, Shahdol, Shivpuri, Sidhi, Tikamgarh.

Botany: Tall, deciduous trees, with smooth, white-grey bark. Leaves silky tomentose when young. Flowers 2-5 in a head, yellow to pinkish- yellow. Fruits orbicular, glabrous, with entire wings.

Flowering & Fruiting: October – June.

Medicinal Parts: Root, bark, fruits.

Chemical constituents: Seed contain Protein.

Leaves contain Phenol, Carboxylic acid, Saponin, Amino acids, Sugars.

Stem bark contain Shikimic acid, quinic acid, fructose, alanine, phenylalanine, tannins. Saponins.

Sap wood contain Quinic acid, glucose, phenylalanine, ellagic acid.

Heart wood containQuercetin, myricetin, glucose, ellagic acid, gallic acid, phenylalanine.

Folk Use: Cold, Cough, Snake bite

Use in literature: Bark – Anaemia, erysepelas, piles, skin diseases, urinary discharges.

33. *Anthocephalus cadamba* (Roxb.) Miq. (Rubiaceae)

Syn.: *A. chinensis* Lam; *A. indicus* A. Rich.

Vern.: Kadam.

Distribution: Mandla, Rewa, Satna.

Botany: A large tree with spreading branches; leaves elliptic-oblong, glabrous above; flowers sweet scented, fruits fleshy.

Flowering & Fruiting: June – September.

Medicinal Parts: Stem Bark.

Chemical constituents: Leaves contain Alkaloid (Kadambine & 3 – œ- di – hydrocadambine); Glycosides alkaloids (Iso – dihydrocadambine & β- Sitosterol).

Root & stem bark contain Quinovic acid, Pentacyclic triterpenic acid, cadambagenic, quinioric acid, saponin.

Flower contain Essential oils.

Folk Use: Rheumatism.

Use in literature: Bark – Cough, debility, diarrhoea, dyspepsia, fever, inflammation, ulcers, vomiting, wound.

Leaves – Ulcers, wounds.

Fruits – Fever.

343. *Aristolochia bracteolata* Lam. (Aristolochiaceae)

Vern.: Kidamar.

Distribution: In wastelands. Bhopal, Shivpuri.

Botany: Perennial prostrate herbs, with purple flowers and capsule fruits. Flowering & Fruiting: September-March.

Medicinal Parts: Roots, Seed.

Chemical constituents: Leaves contain Ceryl alcohol, β-Sitosterol, Aristolochic acid, KCl.

Roots contain Aristolochic acid, KCl, KNO_3.

Folk Use: Fever, Intestinal worms

Use in literature: Roots & Leaves – Amenorrhoea, boils, colic, constipation, dysmenorrhoea, dyspepsia, eczema, inflammations, intsestinal worms, gonorrhoea, skin diseases, syphilis.

35. *Aristolochia indica* L. (Aristolochiaceae)

Syn.: *A. lanceolata* Wight.

Vern.: Isarmul.

Distribution: In mixed forests. Chhatarpur.

Botany: Twining, woody herbs, with elliptic-ovate or obovate-panduriform leaves. Flowers greenish-white, in axillary racemes. Capsules oblong-globose; seeds winged.

Flowering & Fruiting: July-February.

Medicinal Parts: Leaves.

Chemical constituents: Plant contains Three bases of Arisotolochine, Nitrogenous acids (Aristinic acid, Aristidinic acid & Aristolic acid); Volatile oil.

Folk Use: Fever

Use in literature: Amenorrhoea, erysepelas, fever, flatulence, rheumatism, scorpion sting, snakebite, spider bite, strangury, ulcer, worms.

36. *Argemone mexicana* L. (Papaveraceae)

Vern.: Satyanashi.

Distribution: In waste places. Common throughout the State.

Botany: Prickly herbs, with yellow sap and pinnatifid and spiny leaves. Flowers yellow, solitary terminal. Capsule prickly.

Flowering & Fruiting: February-June.

Medicinal Parts: Leaves,Root, Seed, Yellow latex.

Chemical constituents: Root contains Berbetine, Protopine nitrate, Betasterol, fatty acids, ceryl alcohol, Allocryptopine.

Flowers contain Tannin, Resin, Argemone oil.

Leaves contain Glucosides, Kampferin, Anthraquinone, essential oil & Chrysophanic acid.

Seeds contain tasteless oil of dark brown colour, Carbohydrates, Albumin, Phosphate, sulphate.

Folk Use: Conjunctivitis, Ringworm, Skin diseases

Use in literature: Root – Skin diseases.

Seed – Diarrhoea, dysentery.

37. *Argyreia speciosa Sweet.* (Convolvulaceae)

Syn.: *A. nervosa* (Burm. f.) Bojer.

Vern.: Samander kapat

Distribution: Rare. Hoshangabad.

Botany: White tomentose twiners, with ovate-cordate leaves, tomentose beneath. Flowers rose-purple and white.

Flowering & Fruiting: April-September.

Medicinal Parts: Root.

Chemical constituents: Plant contains Arginine, Lycine, Valine, Behenic acid, Linolic acid, linolenic acid, Oleic acid, Argoclavine, Clanoclavine–I & II, Elymoclavine, Ergine, Isoergine, Ergometrine, fastuclavine, Isosetoclavin, setoclavine, Lysergine, Lysergol, Lysergic acid, Caffeic acid, Anthocyanin, Cumarine, Flavonoids, Quercetine, Kaempferol, β- Setosterol.

Folk Use: Rheumatism

Use in literature: Leaf – Eczema, itching, ringworm, skin diseases.

Root – Gonorrhoea, rheumatism, syphilis.

38. *Asparagus racemosus* Willd. (Liliaceae)

Syn.: *A. javanica* Kunth.; *A. sarmentosus* Graham.

Vern.: Shataveri.

Distribution: Throughout the State.

Botany: Scandent, spinous undershrubs, with faciculated tuberous roots. Leaves absent, branches modified into linear, leaf-like cladodes. Flowers in racemes. Fruits globose.

Flowering & Fruiting: August-January.

Medicinal Parts: Fleshy roots.

Chemical constituents: Fleshy roots contain Sugars, mucilage & saponins.

Folk Use: Rheumatism, Tonic, Typhoid

Use in literature: Root – Biliousness, diseases of the blood & the eye, dysentery, epilepsy, inflammation, leprosy, night blindness, throat complaint, tuberculosis, tumour.

39. *Azadirachta indica* A. Juss. (Meliaceae)

Syn.: *Melia azadirachta* L.

Vern.: Neem.

Distribution: Almost throughout the State. Commonly Planted.

Botany: Evergreen trees, with serrate or crenate, 7-17 leaflets and white flowers in panicles. Drupes ovoid, yellow when ripe.

Flowering & Fruiting: March – May.

Medicinal Parts: Whole plant, root bark, stem bark, leaves, flowers, fruits.

Chemical constituents: Plant contains Margocin, Nimbadin, Sulphur, Nimban, Nimbosterol, Tannin, essential oil, Resin, Glycosides, Fatty acids, gum, free amino acids.

Leaves contain Quercetin, β- Sitosterol (Nimbasterol).

Folk Use: Ascariasis, Chiken pox, Fever, Measles, Scabies, Skin diseases, Urticaria

Use in literature: Stem bark – Burning sensation, fever, itching, skin diseases, Ulcer, urinary disorders.

Leaves – Diseases of the eye, fever, inflammation, skin diseases, ulcer, urinary disorders.

40. *Bacopa monnieri* (L.) Penn. (Scrophulariaceae)

Syn.: *Herpestis monnieri* (L.) H. B. & K.; *Moniera cuneifolia* Michx.; *Gratiola monniera* L.

Vern.: Brahmi.

Distribution: In marshy and swampy area. Chhatarpur, Damoh, Dhar, Gwalior, Mandla, Panna, Rewa, Shivpuri, Sidhi, W. Nimar.

Botany: A prostrate gregarious herb with spreading or ascending branches, rooting at the nodes. Leaves sessile, decussate, obovate-oblong or spathulate, succulent. Flowers axillary, solitary on slender pedicels. Corolla bluish –purplish; anthers bluish-purple. Capsules ovoid, glabrous.

Flowering & Fruiting: July-April.

Medicinal Parts: Whole plant.

Chemical constituents: Plant contains Alkaloids – Brahmine & Herpestine, Bacoside A & B (Saponins), Betulic acid, Hersaponin, Nicotine, Becogenin – A, Potassium, Sodium, Calcium, Iron, Oleic acid, Palmitic acid.

Folk Use: Fever.

Use in literature: Blood diseases, cough, debility after heart attack, dyspepsia, epilepsy, fever, hoarsness of voice, insomnia, less memory, tension.

41. *Balanites aegyptiaca* (L.) Del. (Simaroubaceae)

Syn.: *B. rouxburghii* Planch.; *Ximenia aegyptiaca* L.

Vern.: Hingot.

Distribution: Gwalior, Satna.

Botany: Spinous trees or shrubs, with 2-foliolate leaves. Flowers greenish-yellow, in axillary fascicled cymes. Fruits oblong, rind hard.

Flowering & Fruiting: October-August.

Medicinal Parts: Fruits, seeds.

Chemical constituents: Fruits & seeds contain Oil of yellow colour and tasteless.

Pulp & fruit contains Saponin.

Folk Use: Worm infestation.

Use in literature: Fruits – Cough, leprosy, skin diseases, ulcer, wound, worm infestation.

Leaf – Cough, throat infection.

42. *Baliospermum montanum* (Willd.) Muell-Arg. (Euphorbiaceae)

Syn.: *B. polyandrum* Wight.; *B. axillare* Blume.

Distribution: Common in shady places and along the bank of drains in mixed forests. Damoh, E. Nimar, Hosahangabad, Indore, Mandla, Narsimhapur, Panna, Rewa, Satna, Seoni, Sidhi.

Botany: An undershrub; with herbaceous branches from roots; leaves variable in shape & size; flowers small, greenish, monoecious in axillary racemes; fruits capsules.

Flowering & Fruiting: February-April.

Medicinal Parts: Seed oil.

Chemical constituents: Root contains 5 new phorbol esters belonging to diterpene hydrocarbotigliane skeleton viz. montain, balliospermin etc.

Leaves contain β-sitosterol, glucosides, hexacosanol.

Folk Use: Rheumatism

Use in literature: Roots – Anaemia, constipation, dropsy, fever, flatulence, haemorrhoids, jaundice, leprosy, leucoderma, skin diseases, strangury, wounds.

Seeds – Flatulence, inflammations.

43. *Barleria prionitis* L. (Acanthaceae)

Vern.: Jhinti.

Distribution: Common as undergrowth in mixed forests. Bhopal, Chhatarpur, Damoh, Gwalior, Hosahangabad, Indore, Jabalpur, Morena, Panna, Raisen, Rewa, Sagar, Seoni, Shivpuri, Sidhi, Tikamgarh.

Botany: Armed undershrubs, with elliptic or ovate-elliptic leaves and yellow flowers in dense spikes. Calyx-lobes glandular. Capsules 4-seeded.

Flowering & Fruiting: September-April.

Medicinal Parts: Root, Seed.

Chemical constituents: Plant contains Beta- Sitosterol, Scutellarein – 7 Rhamocyl Glucoside, Iridoids, Barlerin and Ac- Barlerin.

Folk Use: Dental trouble, Fever, Snake bite

Acrid, Anti-inflammatory, Antiseptic, Appetiser, bitter, diaphoretic, diuretic, expectorant, heating.

Use in literature: Leaf juice- Abdominal disorders, catarrha, fever.

Dried bark – Cough.

Decoction of plant – Cough, dropsy, Paralysis, toothache.

Paste of root – is applied on boils & glandular swelling.

44. *Bauhinia purpurea* L. (Caesalpiniaceae)

Vern.: Kaliar.

Distribution: On roadsides and in mixed forests. Balaghat, Bhopal, Damoh, Gwalior, Indore, Jabalpur, Seoni, Sidhi.

Botany: Tree; branches stout, glaberescent; leaves roundish, divided half way down into 2 obtuse lobes; flowers fragrant in terminal and axillary few flowered racemes; pods subwoody, flat pointed at both ends, glabrous; seeds 12-16, oblong-ellipsoid, brown.

Flowering & Fruiting: September – November.

Medicinal Parts: Stem bark.

Chemical constituents: Flower contains Pelargonidin–3–glucoside, Pelargonidin – 3 – Triglucoside, Chalcon galactoside, Isoquercetin and Astragalin.

Folk Use: Oral ulcer.

Use in literature: Flower – Blood dysentery, piles.

Stem bark – Diarrhoea.

Root bark – Cough, goitre, haemorroids, leucoderma.

45. *Bauhinia racemosa Lam.* (Caesalpiniaceae)

Syn.: *Piliostigma racemosa* (Lamk.) Bentham.

Distribution: In sal and mixed forests and roadsides. Balaghat, Chhatarpur, Chhindwara, Damoh, E. Nimar, Gwalior, Jabalpur, Hoshangabad, Mandla, Panna, Rewa, Sagar, Satna, Seoni, Shahdol, Shivpuri, Sidhi.

Botany: Deciduous trees.bark grey, rough. Leaves broader than longer. Flowers in terminal, leaf opposed racemes, creamy-white. Pods falcate, turgid. Seeds oval, black.

Medicinal Parts: Stem bark, leaves.

Chemical constituents: Stem bark contains Octacosane, B-amyrin, B-sitosterol.

Seeds- Protein, pentosan, mucilage.

Folk Use: Diarrhoea, Dysentery, Headache, Malaria fever

Use in literature: Root bark- Diarrhoea, dysentery, inflammation, skin diseases, ulcers.

Stem bark, Leaves- Biliousness, diseases of blood, fistula, headache, urinary discharges.

Flowers- Cough, haemorrhages, piles.

46. *Bauhinia variegata* L. (Caesalpiniaceae)

Vern.: Kachnar.

Distribution: In mixed forests. Balaghat, Bhopal, Chhindwada, W. Nimar, Indore, Mandla, Seoni, Shahdol, Shivpuri.

Botany: Medium-sized deciduous trees. Leaves orbicular, 2-lobed. Flowers white to pink. Pods flat, glabrous, brown.

Flowering & Fruiting: August– February.

Medicinal Parts: Stem bark.

Chemical constituents: Stem bark contains Sugar & Tannins.

Flowers contain Octacosanol, β- stiosterol, flavinoid.

Seeds & bark contain Myrcetol, glycoside, kaempferol, glucoside.

Folk Use: Diarrhoea, Dysentery, Piles, Worms

Use in literature: Bark – Asthma, blood diseases, dysmenorrhoea, leprosy, leucoderma, stomach trouble, tuberculous glands, ulcers, wound.

Flowers – Blood diseases, bronchitis, headache, vaginal discharges.

47. *Blumea lacera* (Burm. f.) DC. (Asteraceae)

Syn.: *B. balsamifera* DC.; *B. densiflora* Hook. f.

Distribution: Common along the road sides, open fields and edges, on moist shaded places. Hosahangabad, Sagar, Seoni, Sidhi.

Botany: A herbaceous erect annual with a strong odour of turpentine; flowers yellow, numerous in heads, both terminal and axillary; fruits achenes, crowned with white pappus hairs.

Flowering & Fruiting: November-January.

Medicinal Parts: Plant.

Chemical constituents: The plant contains acetylenic compounds, Diester of Coniferol alcohol, Thiophenen derivatives, Campesterol, hentriacontane, Hentriaceontanol, α-amyrin and its acetate, Lupeol and its acetate, β-sitosterol.

Folk Use: Antiseptic, Earache, Pneumonia

Use in literature: Plant – Burning sensation, bronchitis, cough, fever, inflammation, intestinal worms, leucorrhoea, liver disorders, wounds.

48. *Boerhavia diffusa* L. (Nyctaginaceae)

Syn.: *B. repens* L.

Vern.: Punarnava.

Distribution: Common along roadsides, river banks and in wastelands. Chhatarpur, Damoh, E. Nimar, Indore, Seoni, Tikamgarh, W. Nimar.

Botany: Decumbent or diffuse, perennial, extensive herbs. Leaves unequal, ovate-oblong. Flowers rose or pink, in panicles or subcapitate umbels. Fruits clavate, 5-ribbed, covered with stalked glandular hairs.

Flowering & Fruiting: October-April.

Medicinal Parts: Root, leaves.

Chemical constituents: Plant contains Alkaloids – Punarnavan, Sterol, β- Sitosterol, œ- Sitosterol, Elentine, Stearic acid, Palmitic acid, Minerals, potassium nitrate, sodium & sulphate & chloride.

Folk Use: Jaundice, Kideny trouble, Snake bite, Typhoid

Use in literature: Anaemia, asthma, biliousness, blood impurities, bronchitis, cough, epilepsy, eye trouble, heart diseases, inflammation, Jaundice.

49. *Bombax ceiba* L. (Bombacaceae)

Syn.: *B. malabaricum* DC.; *Salmalia malabarica* (DC.) Schott. & Endl.

Vern.: Semal.

Distribution: Damoh, Jabalpur, Sagar, Seoni, Sidhi.

Botany: Deciduous trees, with prickly trunk and digitately 5 to 7-foliolate leaves. Flowers crimson or yellow, crowded at the end of leafless branches. Capsules woody, 5-valved.

Flowering & Fruiting: February – May.

Medicinal Parts: Root, Stembark.

Chemical constituents:

Seed contains Hexacosanol, tocopherol, terenes.

Bark contains Lupeol, B- sitosterol.

Root contains Triacontanol, B- sitosterol.

Flowers (Petals) contain Essential oil, Hentriacontane, Hentriacontanol, Quercetin, Kaempferol, B- sitosterol.

Folk Use: Dysentery, Prompte conception, Wound

Medicinal Uses: Root – Biliousness, Inflammation.

Flower – Blood purifier, leucorrhoea.

Fruits- Leprosy.

Gum – blood diseases, diarrhoea, dysentery, leucorrhoea, monorrhagia.

50. *Borassus flabellifer* L. (Arecaceae)

Syn.: *B. flabelliformis* Roxb.

Distribution: Cultivated. Dhar, Jabalpur.

Botany: A very tall, erect, magnificient dioecious palms; leaves 1-1.5m diam with 60-80 segments, folded along midrib; edges of petioles spinose; spadices very large; drupes large subglobose.

Medicinal Parts: Leaves.

Chemical constituents: Stem juice contains Minerals like iron; protein, sucrose, glucose, thiamin, riboflavin, nicotinic acid, vitamin C.

Folk Use: Burning sensation during urination

Use in literature: Root – Burning sensation, inflammations. Strangury.

Fruits – Burning sensation, colic, constipation, dyspepsia, flatulence, intestinal worms, leprosy, skin diseases.

51. *Boswellia serrata* Roxb. ex Colebr. (Burseraceae)

Syn.: *B. glabra* Roxb.

Vern.: Salai.

Distribution: Bhopal, Rewa, Seoni, Shahdol.

Botany: Deciduous tree, with bark peeling off in this flakes. Leaves imparipinnate, 7 to many-foliolate. Flowers white, bisexual. Drupes trigonous.

Flowering & Fruiting: February- April.

Medicinal Parts: Bark, gum-resin.

Chemical constituents: Bark contains Carbohydrates, Glucosides and β-sitosterol.

Gum resin contains Diterpine, alcohol, serratol, β-boswellic acid, essential oil.

Folk Use: Dysentery, Rheumatism, Stomachache

Use in literature: Bark – Asthma, dysentery, skin diseases, ulcers.

Gum-resin – Arthritis, asthma, bronchitis, cough, dysentery, fevers, jaundice, stomachache, syphilis.

52. *Brassica nigra* (L.) Koch. (Brassicaceae)

Syn.: *Sinapis nigra* L.; *S. erysimoides* Roxb.

Vern.: Banarasi Rai.

Distribution: In Cultivated. Indore.

Botany: A rigid, Branching annual upper leaves entire. Flowers bright yellow, in nacked racemes. Fruits siliqua. Flowering & Fruiting: December-March.

Medicinal Parts: Seeds.

Chemical Constituents: Seed contains Glucoside Singirin, Sinapine & a Volatile Isothiocyanate and Essential oil.

Folk Use: Headache

Use in literature: Seeds – Anthelmintic, Appetiser, Cough, Enlargement of spleen, Itching, Skin diseases, Tumours.

53. *Brassica campestris* L. (Brassicaceae)

Vern.: Sarson

Distribution: Very largely grown during the cold season in rotation with other crops.

Botany: Annual erect herbs; leaves lyrate-sinuate to lanceolate. Flowers in oblong corymbs, elongating into racemes. Petals clawed, yellow. Fruits siliqua.

Flowering & Fruiting: January-April.

Medicinal Parts: Seed oil, Fruit.

Chemical constituents: The seeds contain glycosinolates.

Folk Use: Cold, Influenza, Snake bite

Use in literature: Cold, Influenza, Fever.

54. *Bridelia retusa* Spreng. (Euphorbiaceae)

Syn.: *B. spinosa* Willd.

Vern.: Ekdania.

Distribution: Common in mixed forests & along roadsides. Balaghat, Bhopal, Chhattarpur, Damoh, Dhar, Hosahangabad, Indore, Mandla, Panna, Satna, Seoni, Shahdol.

Botany – A shrub or a tree up to 18 m in height with 7 cm. long, strong conical spine. Flowering & Fruiting: July-February.

Medicinal parts – Stem, Bark.

Chemical constituents:

Fruit pulp – β-Sitosterol, Gallic acid, Ellagic acids.

Seeds – Ellagic acid.

Bark – Triterpenoid Ketone, Tannin.

Folk Use: Gum trouble, Rheumatism, Toothache

55. *Buchanania lanzan* Spreng. (Anacardiaceae)

Vern.: Chironji.

Distribution: Very common in dry deciduous forests. Balaghat, Bhopal, Hosahangabad, Indore, Jabalpur, Mandla, Rewa, Sagar, Satna, Seoni, Shivpuri, Tikamgarh.

Botany: Tall trees, with straight trunk, leaves elliptic-oblong. Flowers greenish-white, in pyramidal panicles. Drupes obiliquely lentiform, smooth, one-seeded.

Flowering & Fruiting: January-June.

Medicinal Parts: Fruits, Leaves.

Chemical constituents: Leaves contain Kaempferol glucoside, quercetain, gallic acid.

Fruit Kernel contains Proteins; minerals as Calcium, phosphorus, iron, magnessium, sodium, copper, potassium, sulpher, chlorine, thiamine, niacin, riboflavin, vitamin C.

Folk Use: Diarrhoea, Mouth eruption

Use in literature:

Roots – Diarrhoea, leprosy, skin diseases.

Leaf – Bronchitis, burning sensation, constipation, cough, dyspepsia, flatulence, leprosy, skin diseases.

Fruits – Asthma, burning sensation, cardiac debility, constipation, cough, fever, inflammations, leprosy, skin diseases, ulcers.

56. *Butea monosperma* (Lamk.) Taub. (Papilionaceae)

Syn.: *B. frondosa* Koenig ex Roxb.

Vern.: Palash.

Distribution: In Sal and mixed forests and Wastelands. Balaghat, Bhopal, Chhatarpur, Damoh, Hosahangabad, Indore, Jabalpur, Mandla, Rewa, Sagar, Seoni, Shahdol, Shivpuri, Sidhi, W. Nimar.

Botany: Medium-sized trees, with 3-foliolate large leaves and orange, showy flowers in racemes. Pods grey-silky.

Flowering & Fruiting: March – June.

Medicinal Parts: Bark, flowers, leaves, seeds, gum.

Chemical constituents: Plant contains Fats, oils, Mucilage, protein, Resin, Butin, Glucoside, Butein, Isomonospermoside, Coreopsin, Sulphruein, Palastirin, butrin, Isobutrin.

Gum contains Thiamine, Riboflavin, fatty acids, myristi acid, palmitic & stearic acid.

Folk Use: Anthelmintic, Asthma, Bodyache, Colic pain, Diarrhoea, Dysentery, Snake bite, Urinary troubles

Use in literature: Root – Elephantiasis, nightblindness.

Bark – Bone fractures, dysentery, hydrocele, piles, tumour, ulcer.

Leaf – Eye diseases

Gum – Cough, dysentery, stomach troubles.

Flower – Burning sensation, eye diseases, gout, leprosy, skin diseases, strangury.

Fruits – Abdominal pain, piles, scorpion sting, skin diseases, tumours, urinary discharges.

Seed – Abdominal pain, piles, scorpion sting, skin diseases, tumours, urinary discharges.

57. *Caesalpinia bonduc* (L.) Taub. (Caesalpiniaceae)

Syn.: *C. bonducella* Fleming.; *C. crista* L.; C. nuga Ait. f.; *Guilandina bounducella* L.

Vern.: Kantak karanj.

Distribution: On forest edges and roadsides. Damoh, Indore, Jabalpur, Mandla, Ratlam, Rewa, Sagar, Seoni, Shivpuri, Sidhi, Tikamgarh.

Botany: Armed shrubs, pinnae 6-8 pairs, with a pair of hooked stipular spines; leaflets 6-9 pairs, elliptic-oblong, obtuse. Racemes often panicled; pods shortly stalked, oblong, densely armed on the faces with wiry prickles, 1-2 seeded.

Flowering & Fruiting**:** June – February.

Medicinal Parts: Root, leaves, seeds.

Chemical constituents: Seed contains Fatty oils, starch, sucrose, caesalpins, bonducellin, fatty acids, phytosterinin, saponins, phytosterols, amino acids, a bitter glucoside- bonducin.

Folk Use: Stomach pain

Use in literature: Leaf – Elephantiasis, small pox.

Fruit – Leucorrhoea, piles, urinary discharges, wounds.

Seed **–** Colic, hydrocele, inflammation, leprosy, malaria, skin diseases.

58. *Cajanus cajan (*L.) Millsp. (Papilionaceae)

Syn.: *C. indicus* Spreng.

Vern.: Arahar.

Distribution: In Cultivation. Bhopal, Indore, Jabalpur, Mandla, Ratlam, Sagar, Shahdol, Shivpuri, Sidhi.

Botany: An erect shrub. Leaflets 3, oblong-lanceolate. Flowers yellow, in corymbose racemes. Pods narrowed at the ends, torulose. Flowering & Fruiting: August-March.

Medicinal Parts: Leaves.

Chemical Constituents: Leaves contain n-Alkanes, Simple esters, Free alcohols, Lupeol, Phytosterols as β-Sitostrerol, Stigmasterol, Campesterol, Cholesterol; Isoflavone as Cajanol; Salicylic acid, Linoleic acid, Oleic acid.

Folk Use: Cuts

Use in literature: Leaves / Seeds – Bronchitis, Cardiac diseases, Cough, Fever, Haemorrhoids, Intestinal Worms, Tumours, Vomiting.

59. *Calotropis gigantea* (L.) Ait. f. (Asclepiadaceae)

Vern.: Safed aak.

Distribution: Common in wastelands and along bundh of cultivated fields. Chhatarpur, Damoh, Hosahangabad Mandla, Seoni, Shahdol.

Botany: Shrubs or small trees, with elliptic-oblong or obovate-oblong leaves. Corolla-buds ovoid; corona-lobes hairy, shorter than staminal column.

Flowering & Fruiting: March-May.

Medicinal Parts: Root, Leaves, Flowers, Milk.

Chemical constituents: Plant contains Mudarol, akundarol, uscharidin calotropin, frugoside, calotroposides – A to G, calotroplupenyl acetate- A, leupeol acetate – B, gigantursenyl acetate – A, gigantursenyl acetate – B.

Folk Use: Asthma, Dog bite, Rheumatism, Whooping cough

Use in literature: Plant – Diseases of the spleen, the liver, the abdomen, Leprosy, leucoderma, piles, tumour, ulcer.

Root bark – Asthma, syphilis.

Flower – Ascites, inflammation, tumour.

Milk – Ascites, diseases of the abdomen, leucoderma, tumour.

60. *Calotropis procera* (Ait.) R. Br. (Asclepiadaceae)

Vern.: Aak.

Distribution: Common in wastelands, along bundh of cultivated fields and roadsides. Balaghat, Chhatarpur, Damoh, Hosahangabad, Jabalpur, Panna, Rewa, Sagar, Satna, Seoni, Shahdol, Sidhi.

Botany: Shrubs or small trees, with ovate or ovate-oblong leaves. Corolla-buds hemispherical; corona-lobes glabrous, equalling or longer than staminal column.

Flowering & Fruiting: Throughout the year.

Medicinal Parts: Root, leaves, flowers, latex.

Chemical constituents: Plant contains Cardiac steroid glycoside-terpenoids, resin, glycosides, carbohydrates, aluminium, Iron, magnesium, sodium.

Folk Use: Asthma, Backache, Fever, Leprosy, Rheumatism, Snake bite, Swelling, Whooping cough

Use in literature: Asthma, cough, dropsy, eczema, inflammation, piles, rheumatism, stranguary, ulcer.

61. *Cannabis sativa* L. (Cannabinaceae)

Vern.: Bhang.

Distribution: Ocasionally in wastelands and along roadsides near habitations, Chhatarpur, Indore.

Botany: Dioecious, aromatic, woody herbs with 3 to 9- foliolate leaves. Flowers white or cream, males in panicels, female's axillary, solitary forming spikes.

Flowering & Fruiting: March-November.

Medicinal Parts: Leaves, the part of male flowering twig resin.

Chemical constituents: Plant contains Cannabinoids, cannabispirans, alkaloids, cannabig lendol, cannabidiolic acid, resin (Cannabinone), gum, sugars, calcium, phosphate, and volatile oil.

Folk Use: Asthma, Diarrhoea

Use in literature: Leaves – Anthelmintic, cuts, ear trouble, skin diseases, wounds.

Flowers – Diarrhoea, dysnetery, gonorrhoea.

62. *Canscora decussate* (Roxb.) Schult. (Gentianaceae)

Vern.: Sankhaphuli.

Distribution: Along roadsides in open forests. Hosahangabad.

Botany: Dichotomously branched annual, with quadrangular Stem and White flowers. Flowering & Fruiting: September-October.

Medicinal Parts: Whole plant.

Chemical Constituents: Loliolide, Triterpenes as Glucose Conscoradione, Friedelin, Canscoridine, Sterols as-Sitosterol, Stigmasterol, Campesterol.

Folk Use: Nervous debility.

Use in literature: Plant – Abdominal disorders, Ascites, Epilepsy, General debility, Inflammation, Intestinal worms, Leprosy, Leucoderma, Nervous debility, Skin diseases, Tuberculosis, Ulcers.

63. *Capparis decidua* (Forsk.) Edgew. (Capparidaceae)

Vern.: Karer.

Distribution: In drier areas. Gwalior, Indore, Shivpuri.

Botany: Leafless spiny shrubs or small trees, with red or Orange-Red flowers in corymbose racemes or fascicles. Berries subglobose, scarlet when ripe.

Flowering & Fruiting: March-July.

Medicinal Parts: Stem.

Chemical constituents: Isothiocyanate glucoside, glucocapparin, stachydrine, n-triaconate, β-carotene, β-sitotsterol, n-triacontanol, n-pentacosane, phthalic acid.

Folk Use: Dental pain.

Use in literature: Root – Amenorrhoea, arthritis, asthma, boils, constipation, cough, dysmenorrhoea, dyspepsia, eruptions, flatulence, gout, hiccough, intestinal worms, lumbago, swelling, vomiting.

Fruits – Cardiac disorders.

64. *Capparis zeylanica* L. (Capparidaceae)

Syn.: *C. horrida* L. f.

Vern.: Ardanda.

Distribution: In dry deciduous forests and roadsides. Balaghat, Indore, Jabalpur, Mandla, Rewa, Satna, Sagar.

Botany: Climbing shrubs; leaves ovate or oblong, entire; stipular spines hooked; petals densely hairy inside; berries subglobose, reddish-brown, with woody pericarp; seeds subglobose. Flowering & Fruiting: January-June.

Medicinal Parts: Root Bark, Leaves, Fruits.

Chemical Constituents: An alkaloid- Phytosterol, Mucilaginous Substance and water soluble acid, L-Stachydrine, Rutin and β-Sitosterol.

Seeds / Leaves – Thioglucoside, Glucocapparin, n-Tricontane & Fixed oil.

Folk Use: Constipation, Stomach pain

Use in literature: Root Bark – Colic.

65. *Capsicum annuum* L. (Solanaceae)

Syn.: *C. longum* DC.; *C. grossum* Willd.; *C. condiforme* Mill.

Vern.: Lal mirch.

Distribution: Cultivated throughout the State as cash crop. Bhopal, Chhatarpur, Damoh.

Botany: Perennial herbs, with lanceolate leaves, white flowers & slender, Green red or orange fruits.

Flowering & Fruiting: Throughout the year.

Medicinal Parts: Fruits, Root.

Chemical constituents: Fruits contain A volatile alkaloid-capsicin; a crystalline substance-capsacin; a volatile oil-solanine; fatty acid, resin.

Folk Use: Fever, Snake bite

Use in literature: Fruits – Arthritis, cholera, cough, dropsy, dyspepsia, fever, flatulence, gout, hoarseness, sciatica.

66. *Cardiospermum halicacabum* L. (Sapindaceae)

Vern.: Kanphuta.

Distribution: Climbing on bushes and hedges along roadsides, forest-clearings, grasslands and in dry deciduous forests. Also common in cultivated fields. Balaghat, Betul, Chhatarpur, Damoh, E. Nimar, Guna, Gwalior, Hosahangabad, Indore, Jabalpur, Jhabua, Mandla, Sagar, Satna, Seoni, Tikamgarh.

Botany: Herbaceous climbers, with 5-fid axillary tendrils and bi-or trinate leaves. Flowers white, in cymes on terminal tendrils.

Flowering & Fruiting: Throughout the year.

Medicinal Parts: Roots, Leaves, Seeds.

Chemical constituents: Seed – Cyanogenic glycoside, essential oil.

Folk Use: Rheumatism

Use in literature: Root – Menorrhoea, arthritis, fever, lumbago, strangury.

Leaves – Arthritis.

Seeds – Arthritis, fever.

67. *Careya arborea* Roxb. (Borringtoniaceae)

Distribution: Growing on hill slopes and along the sides of streams. Balaghat, Mandla, Seoni, Sidhi.

Botany: A small to medium sized deciduous tree with yellowish-white flowers and berries fruit.

Flowering & Fruiting: March-July.

Medicinal Parts: Bark, leaves, flowers, fruits.

Folk Use: Cold, Cough, Fever, Joint pain

Use in literature: Bark – Bronchitis, catarrh, colic, cough,dysentery, dyspepsia, leucoderma, tumours.

Fruit – Dyspepsia.

68. *Carica papaya* L. (Caricaceae)

Vern.: Papita.

Distribution: Commonly cultivated, almost throughout State.

Botany: A rapidly growing tree, up to 7 m. tall, with milky sap. Leaves palmately-lobed and flowers creamy yellow; female flowers in short clusters and males in long drooping panicles.

Flowering & Fruiting: Almost throughout the year.

Medicinal Parts: Fruits, Latex.

Chemical constituents: Fruits pulp contains Sucrose, invert sugar, papain, malic acid, salts of tartaric acid & citric acid, pectins, carotenoid, vitamins.

Latex contains Enzymes papain & chymopapain.

Folk Use: Dyspepsia.

Use in literature: Fruits – Bronchitis, cough, dyspepsia, inflammations, intestinal worms, psoriasis, ringworm, skin diseases.

Latex – Amenorrhoea, constipation, dysmenorrhoea, dyspepsia, leprosy, skin diseases.

69. *Carissa carandas* L. (Apocynaceae)

Syn.: *C. cognesta* Wt.

Vern.: Karonda.

Distribution: Common along the edges of forests also under cultivation. Damoh, Jabalpur, Sagar.

Botany: Erect or scandent shrubs, with paired spines at each node. Leaves elliptic-oblong to ovate. Flowers white, in corymbose cymes. Berries elliptic oblong, fleshy. Flowering & Fruiting: May October.

Medicinal Parts: Leaves, Root, Fruits.

Chemical Constituents: Root contain – β-sitosterol, a Sesquiterpene as Carissone: a Lignancarinol, Odoroside-H, Digitoxigenin, Glucose, D-digitalose, Lupeol, Ursolic acid, Methyl ursolate.

Fruits contain – Triterpene alcohol as Carissol, Glucose, Galactose, Serine, Glutamine, Alanine, Valine, Glycine, Carissic acid, Phenylalanine.

Folk Use: Scurvy, Stomachache

Use in literature: Roots – Intestinal worms, Pruritus, Scabies, Stomach disorders.

Ripe fruits – Burning sensation, Skin diseases, Scabies, Pruritus.

Unripe fruits – Anorexia, Diarrhoea, Intermittent fever.

70. *Cassia fistula* L. (Caesalpiniaceae)

Syn.: *C. rhombifolia* Roxb.; *C. excelsa* H. B. & K.

Vern.: Amaltas.

Distribution: In Sal and mixed forests and roadsides. Balaghat, Bhopal, Chhindwada, E. Nimar, Hosahangabad, Indore, Jabalpur, Khandwa, Mandla, Panna, Raisen, Sagar, Satna, Sehore, Seoni, Shahdol, Shivpuri, Sidhi.

Botany: Deciduous tree; branchlets glabrous; leaves eglandular; leaflets 4-8 pairs,ovate, silvery, pubescent beneath when young;

flowers in lax racemes; pods long, cylindrical, nearly straight, smooth, shining, brown-black.

Flowering & Fruiting: March – May.

Medicinal Parts: Leaves, Seed, Fruit.

Chemical constituents: Fruit contains Glycosides, carbohydrates, resin, tannins, magnessium, calcium, potassium, iron & other compounds are fistucacidin, beta-sitosterol, n-tricontanol, leucopelavgonidin, flavonoids, glucosides, gum, and volatile oil.

Folk Use: Rheumatism, Skin diseases, Snake bite

Use in literature: Root – Burning sensation, leprosy, skin disease, syphilis, tuberculous glands.

Bark – Boils, colic, constipation, diabetes, dyspepsia, fever, leprosy, pustules, ringworm.

Leaves – Fever, leprosy, skin disease, ulcers.

Flowers – Burning sensation, bronchitis, cough, pruritus, skin disease.

Fruit – Burning sensation, cardic disorders, colic, fever, gout, inflamation, jaundice, pruritus, rheumatism, Skin disease.

71. *Cassia obtusifolia* L. (Caesalpiniaceae)

Syn.: *C. tora* L.; *C. toroides* Roxb.; *C. foetida* Pers., *Senna tora* (L.) Roxb.

Vern.: Chakunda.

Distribution: Common in Wastelands. Balaghat, Chhindwara, Damoh, E. Nimar, Hosahangabad, Indore, Jabalpur, Mandla, Panna, Raisen, Sagar, Shivpuri, Tikamgarh.

Botany: Suffruticose herbs. With 3 pairs of leaflets and glands between them. Flowers yellow or reddish tinged, geminate; all 7 anthers rounded at apex. Pods linear, turgid.

Flowering & Fruiting: August-April.

Medicinal Parts: Leaves, seeds.

Chemical constituents: Seed contains Glucosides, (Emodin) proteins, steroids, Amino acids, Reducing sugars, Triterpenes,

Tannins, oleic acid, Linotic acid, Palmitic acid, Lignocenic acid, Rubrofusarin, Fixed oils, sodium, Potassium & Iron.

Folk Use: Rheumatism

Use in literature: Leaves & seeds – Bronchitis, cardiac disorders, colic, constipation, cough, dyspepsia, flatulence, intermittent fever, leprosy, pruritus, ringworm, skin diseases.

72. *Cassia sophera* L. (Caesalpiniaceae)

Syn.: *Senna sophera* (L.) Roxb.

Vern.:Kasunda.

Distribution: On edges of mixed forests. Bhopal, Chhattarpur, Mandla, Sagar.

Botany – Shrubs; leaflets 5-10 pairs; flowers yellow; pods turgid. Flowering & Fruiting: November-February.

Medicinal parts – Stem Bark.

Chemical constituents: Emodin and Chrysophani acid.

Seed contain tannic acid, Mucilage, Fatty oil Emodin & a Toxalbumin, Rhamnetin-3-0-B-D Glucoside along with Chrysophanol from flowers.

Folk Use: Diabetes

Use in literature: Leaves – used externally in Ringworm.

Decoction of plant – Used in acute bronchitis.

73. *Catharanthus roseus* Don (Apocynaceae)

Syn.: *Vinca rosea* L.; *Lochnera rosea* Reichb.

Vern.: Sadabahar.

Distribution: Common in sand wastelands and along roadsides. Balaghat, Betul, Chhatarpur, Hosahangabad, Indore, Satna, Seoni, Sidhi.

Botany: An erect herb, with simple opposite leaves; white or rosy flowers.

Flowering & Fruiting: Round the year.

Medicinal Parts: Leaves.

Chemical constituents: Plant contains Indole alkaloids- vincamine; BisIndole alkaloids–vinblastine. Vincristine; Aracidic acid, Behenic acid, Lauric acid, Linolenic acid, oleic acid, palmitic acid, Stearic acid (Seeds).

Stem contains β – Sitosterol, Ursolic acid.

Folk Use: Diabetes

Use in literature: Diabetes, haemorrhagic diseases, leucomea, menorrhagea.

74. *Cayratia carnosa* (Wall.ex Wight) Gagnep. (Vitaceae)

Syn.: *Vitis carnosa* L.; *Vitis trifolia* L.

Vern.: Amal-bel.

Distribution: Balaghat, Damoh, Dhar, Gwalior, Hosahangabad, Indore, Mandla, Panna, Rewa, Sagar, Seoni, Shivpuri, Sidhi.

Botany: Herbaceous climbers, with 3- foliolate leaves and greenish – white flowers in axillary or pseudo, terminal cymes. Berries obovate-globose, dark purple to black when ripe.

Flowering & Fruiting: July – October.

Medicinal Parts: Root.

Folk Use: Dog bite

Use in literature: Cardiac disorders, dropsy, fever, haemorrhoids, neuralgia, splenopathy, strangury, tumors, ulcer, wounds.

75. *Celastrus paniculatus* Willd. (Celastraceae)

Syn.: *C. montana* Roth.; *C. multiflora* Roxb.

Vern.: Malkangani.

Distribution: Balaghat, Damoh, Hosahangabad, Panna, Satna, Seoni, Shivpuri, Sidhi.

Botany: Unarmed, shrubby climbers, with ovate-elliptic leaves and greenish yellow flowers in terminal panicles. Ovary free from the disc.

Flowering & Fruiting: November– February.

Medicinal Parts: Bark, seed oil.

Chemical constituents: Seed contains Concentrate reddish-brownish, bitter and pungent oil, Resin, Tannin, celastrin and paniculatin.

Folk Use: Fever, Leprosy, Leucorrhoea, Rheumatism,

Use in literature: Bark – Brain tonic.

Seed – Abdominal disorders, amenorrhoea, asthma, cardiac debility, dysenorrhoea, fever, inflammation, leucoderma, leprosy, paralysis, pruritus, skin diseases.

76. *Celosia argentea* L. (Amaranthaceae)

Syn.: *C. cristata* L.

Vern.: Safed murga.

Distribution: Common as weed in cultivated fields, wastelands, along roadsides and in dried up river beds. Balaghat, Chhatarpur, Damoh, E. Nimar, Gwalior, Hosahangabad, Indore, Mandla, Panna, Sagar, Satna, Seoni, Shivpuri, Sidhi, Tikamgarh, W. Nimar..

Botany: Erect annuals. Leaves linear-lanceolate or ovate-elliptic. Flowers white or pink. Seeds lenticular, black, shining.

Flowering & Fruiting: August-December.

Medicinal Parts: Root, seeds.

Chemical constituents: Seed contain Saponin of hyaluronic acid.

Folk Use: Diarrhoea, Dysentery, Malaria

Use in literature: Seeds – Diarrhoea, dysuria, seminal diseases.

77. *Centella asiatica* (L.) Urban (Apiaceae)

Syn.: *Hydrocotyle asiatica* L.

Vern.: Mandukaparni.

Distribution: Balaghat, Hosahangabad, Indore, Sidhi.

Botany: Creeping herbs, with broadly suborbicular leaves and pink or red flowers in fasciculate umbels. Fruits ovoid.

Flowering & Fruiting: May – November.

Medicinal Parts: Whole plant.

Chemical constituents: Plant contains Alkaloids-Brahmi, Herpestin, Bacosides A & B In Bacoside-A: Arabnosil, glucose, Arabnose, Becogenine, Betulic acid, D-Manitol, Stigmasterol, β-Sitosterol & Tannins.

Leaves contain Glucoside, Volatile oil.

Dry parts contain Centoic acid, centalic acid.

Whole plant also contains Pectic acid, valerin, resin, ascorbic acid.

Folk Use: Brain tonic, Hypertension

Use in literature: Abdominal disorders, amentia, asthma, bronchitis, cardiac debility, epilepsy, fever, hiccough, hoarseness, insomnia, leprosy, strangury.

78. *Centipeda minima* (L.) A. Br. & Aschers (Asteraceae)

Syn.: *C. orbicularis* Lour.

Distribution: Common in moist places. Damoh, Mandla, Seoni, Sidhi.

Medicinal parts: Leaves, Whole plant.

Chemical constituents:

Plant: Lupeol, Hexacosanol, β-Sitosterol, Stigmasterol, Centipedaoic acid, Flavons.

Folk Use: Swollen gums, Toothache

Use in literature:

Leaf – Leucoderma, Diseases of the Blood and the Skin, Hysteria.

Seed – Headache, Colds in the head, Paralysis, Pains in Joints.

79. *Chenopodium album* L. (Chenopodiaceae)

Vern.: Bathua.

Distribution: Common in cultivated fields, along river banks and in wastelands. Chhatarpur, Damoh, Hosahangabad, Jabalpur, Mandla, Panna, Sagar, Satna, Sidhi.

Botany: Herbs, with oblong-rhomboid, somewhat fleshy leaves. Flowers pale-green, born in clusters in paniculate, ebracteate spikes; perianth-segements without any swelling on the back. Seeds rugose.

Flowering & Fruiting: November – February.

Medicinal Parts: Whole plant, Leaves.

Chemical constituents: Plant contains A volatile oil, which contains Ascaridol; saponin, Vitamin- C, Magnessium, Phosphate, Carotene.

Folk Use: Rheumatism

Use in literature: Cardiac disorders, dyspepsia, flatulence, general debility, helminthiasis, Peptic ulcer, seminal weakness, strangury.

80. *Chlorophytum tuberosum* Bak. (Liliaceae)

Vern.: Safed musli.

Distribution: In Sal forests and in open places among grasses. Hosahangabad.

Botany: Annual herbs, with many cylindric root – fibres ending in ellipsoid tubers. Leaves linear – lanceolate. Flowers white, in dense racemes. Capsules obovoid transversely veined.

Flowering & Fruiting: July – August.

Medicinal Parts: Root, tubers.

Chemical constituents: Root contains Steroids, resin, phenolics, tannins, carbohydrates, calcium, magnessium and potassium.

Folk Use: Aphrodisiac Impotency, Tonic

Use in literature: Root and tuber – Diarrrhoea, dysentery, general debility, gonorrhoea, leucorrhoea, seminal debility.

81. *Chrozophora rottleri* (Geis.) A. Juss. ex Spreng. (Euphorbiaceae)

Syn.: *C. plicata* Hook. F.

Distribution: Common in wastelands, dried ditches, roadsides, river beds & along the railway tract. Damoh, E. Nimar, Mandla.

Botany: Stellately hairy herbs, branched in the upper region. Leaves entire or 3-lobed, ovate to suborbicular. Sepals of female flowers triangular; stigma red. capsules purple. Flowering & Fruiting: March-May.

Medicinal Parts: Root.

Folk Use: Cough

Use in literature: Seeds – Cathartic.

82. *Cicer arietinum* L. (Papilionaceae)

Distribution: Commonly cultivated as a cold weather crop for its seeds used as a pulse. Bhopal, Chhindwara, Hosahangabad, Indore, Mandla, Sagar, Shivpuri, Sidhi.

Botany: Much branched herbs, with pinnate leaves and turgid-oblong fruits.

Flowering & Fruiting: November- March.

Medicinal Parts: Leaves, Seeds.

Chemical constituents: Leaves contain Vanillic, P-hydroxybenzoic acid; oxalic acid, malic acid, arginine, tryosine, lycine, cystine, tryptophane; carotenoids & vitamins.

Folk Use: Jaundice

Use in literature: Leaves – Bronchitis, Dyspepsia.

Seed – Bronchitis, burning sensation, inflammations, leprosy, skin diseases.

83. *Cissampelos pareira* L. (Menispermaceae)

Syn.: *C. hexandra* Roxb.; *C. convolvulacea* Willd.; *C. hernadifolia* Wall.

Vern.: Akauadi.

Description: Along road sides and in the forests. Common throughout the State.

Botany: Twining, dioecious shrubs, with orbicular or reniform leaves, greenish yellow flowers and subglobose fruits which become red on ripening.

Flowering & Fruiting: June-January.

Medicinal Parts: Root, bark.

Chemical constituents: Root & its bark contains Alkaloids, cissampareine, berberine, cissampeline, pelosine, hayantin, hayatinin, saponin.

Folk Use: Bodyache, Cold, Dropsy, Dyspepsia, Fever, Snake bite, Urinary complaints

Use in literature: Plant – Asthma, burning sensation, dysentery, eruptions, fever, heart trouble, itching, piles, skin diseases, ulcers, vomiting.

Root – Conjunctivitis, cough, diarrhoea, dropsy, dyspepsia, scorpion sting, snakebite, stomach pain.

84. *Cissus quadrangularis* L. (Vitaceae)

Syn.: *Vitis quadrangularis* Wall.

Vern.: Hadjor.

Distribution: An extensive climber on hedges or trees.

Botany: A large perennial climber. Stems fleshy cactus – like jointed with quadrangular 4 – winged internodes and a tendril at some of the nodes, leaf – ovate or reniform, and are opposed. Flowers greenish – white in shortly peduncled umbellate cymes. Fruits berry, red when ripe.

Flowering & fruiting: July – August.

Medicinal parts: Whole plant.

Chemical constituents: Plant contains Carotene, calcium oxalate, vitamin – C, alpha-amyrone and β – sitostosterol.

Folk Use: Bone fracture

Use in Literature: Whole plant – Chronic ulcers, colic, convulsions, dyspepsia, epilepsy, flatulence, fractures, haemoptysis, haemorrhages, haemorrhoids, helminthiasis, leprosy, ophthalmopathy, otorrhoea, skin diseases, spanomenorrhea, swellings, tumours.

85. *Citrullus colocynthis* (L.) Schrad. (Cucurbitaceae)

Syn.: *C. vulgaris* Schard.

Vern.: Indrayan.

Botany: Perennial herbs, with 2 to 3-fid tendrils and deeply 3 to 5-lobed leaves. Flowers greenish-yellow. Fruits globose, mottled with yellowish blotches.

Flowering & fruiting: November– January.

Medicinal parts: Root.

Chemical constituents: Root contains Steroid, œ – Elaterin, Colosynthin, Colosynthothin, saponins.

Seed contains Fixed oil, Phytosterolin, Phytosterol, Saponin, Alkaloid, Glycosides, Tannins, Fatty acids.

Fruits contain Citrulluin, Citrullic acid, Glucose, fructose, Manolic acid.

Folk Use: Rheumatism.

Use in Literature: Root – Uteralgia, Mammillitis, Rheumatalgia, Ophthalmia, ascites, jaundice.

Fruits – Ascites, asthma, bronchitis, constipation, dyspepsia, elephantiasis, jaundice, leucoderma, tumours, ulcers.

86. *Citrus limon* (L.) Burm. f. (Rutaceae)

Vern.: Limbu.

Distribution: Bhopal, Damoh, Sagar.

Botany: Thorny trees, with ovate-elliptic leaves, white flowers tinged with pink-purple and oval or oblong fruits.

Flowering & Fruiting: During winters.

Medicinal Parts: Leaves.

Chemical constituents: Oil from peel contains d-limonene, camphene, linalool.

Peel contains Bitter principle, essential oil, hesperidin, citronellal, bergamotine, eriocitrin, apigenin, luteolin, chrysoseriol, quercetin, isorhamnetin, limocitin, limocitriol.

Seeds contain Bitter principles, obacunone, limonin.

Roots contain Xanthyletin, stigmasterol, β-sitosterol.

Folk Use: Swelling of eyes

Use in literature: Fruits – Bronchitis, colic, constipation, cough, dyspepsia, fatigue, flatulence, helminthiasis, scabies, vomiting.

87. *Clematis triloba* Heyne ex Roth. (Ranunculaceae)

Vern.: Murhari.

Distribution: As undergrowth in mixed deciduous forests. Hosahangabad, Narsimhpur.

Botany: An extensive climber, with opposite leaves and white flowers in axillary corymbose panicles. Flowering & Fruiting: October-December.

Medicinal Parts: Roots.

Chemical Constituents: Anemonin, Alcoholic extract of plant is hypotensive and spamolytic.

Folk Use: Snake bite

Use in literature: Leaves – Blood diseases, Syphilis, Scrofula, Leprosy, Chronic fevers, Heart troubles, Boils, Itching.

88. *Cleome gynandra* L. (Cleomaceae)

Syn.: *Gynandropsis gynandra* DC.

Vern.: Hulhul.

Distribution: In Waste lands. Damoh, Gwalior, Jabalpur, Mandla, Sagar, Satna, Sidhi.

Botany: Glandular hairy herbs, with 3 to 5-foliolate leaves. Flowers white, in terminal racemes. Capsules linear-cylindric.

Flowering & Fruiting**:** June – November.

Medicinal Parts: Root, Leaves, seeds.

Chemical constituents: Plant contains Essential oil.

Seed contains Cleomin.

Folk Use: Anthelmintic, Headache, Rheumatism, Skin diseases

Use in literature: Root **–** Ascites, earache, fever, spleen enlargement, tumours, ulcers.

89. *Cleome viscosa* L. (Cleomaceae)

Syn.: *C. icosandra* L.

Vern.: Hulhur.

Distribution: In Waste lands. Balaghat, Dhar, Hosahangabad, Indore, Jabalpur, Mandla, Raisen, Rewa, Satna, Sidhi, Tikamgarh.

Botany: Glandular hariy herbs, with 3 to 5-foliolate leaves. Flowers yellow, in leafy racemes; stamens more than 10. Capsules cylindric, beaked.

Flowering & Fruiting**:** June – September.

Medicinal Parts: Whole plant, Leaves.

Chemical constituents: Seed contain Viscosic acid & visosin.

Folk Use: Boils, Ear trouble, Fever, Vermicide

Use in literature: Root – Otaglia.

Seed – Cardiac disorders, diarrhoea, dyspepsia, fever.

90. *Clerodendrum phlomidis* L. f. (Verbenaceae)

Vern.: Arni.

Distribution: In Wastelands. Chhatarpur, Gwalior, Indore, Panna, Rewa, Sagar, Satna, Shivpuri, W. Nimar.

Botany: Erect or scandent shrubs, with solid stem and opposite, rhomboid – ovate leaves. Flowers white, in panicles. Fruits obovoid.

Flowering & Fruiting: October – February.

Medicinal Parts: Root, Leaves, Flower.

Chemical constituents: Plant contains Pectolinargenin, Scuttelarein, Apigenin, Clerosterol, Hispudilin, Luteolin, Clerodendrin, Cerolic acid, Cerylalcohol, Raffinose, cholesterol, β – Sitosterol.

Folk Use: Earache, Fever, Miscarriage

Use in literature: Root – Anemia, constipation, diabetes, dyspepsia, fever, inflammation, piles, swelling.

91. *Clerodendrum serratum* (L.) Moon. (Verbenaceae)

Syn.: *C. dentatum* Lam.

Vern.: Bharangi.

Distribution: In Sal forests. Balaghat, Damoh, Hosahangabad, Indore, Mandla, Seoni.

Botany: A shrub, usually herbaceous but occasionally woody, with 4-angular stems. Leaves sessile or subsessile, opposite or ternate. Flowers blue, purple or white, 2-lipped, lips unequal. Drupe broadly obovoid, succulent, dark-purple when ripe.

Flowering & Fruiting: August-October.

Medicinal Parts: Roots, leaves.

Chemical constituents: Roots & leaves contain Glycosides, olianolic acid, querteroic acid, serotonic acid, manitol, saponins, orange coloured resinous substance, starch.

Folk Use: Bronchitis, Eye diseases, Snake bite

Use in literature: Root – Asthma, bronchitis, chronic, colic, consumption, cough, dropsy, dyspepsia, flatulence, fever, helminthiasis, hiccough, inflammation, leprosy, leucoderma, nasitis, skin diseases, tumours, tubercular glands.

92. *Clerodendrum viscosum* Vent. (Verbenaceae)

Syn.: *C. infortunatum* Auct.

Vern.: Bhant.

Distribution: Common along roadsides. Damoh, Hosahangabad, Rewa.

Botany – Large tomentose shrubs or small tress; branchlets 4-angled; flowers Pinkish White, in lax terminal panicles; drupe black in enlarged Pink calyx. Flowering & Fruiting: March-June.

Medicinal parts – Leaves, Roots, Inflorescence, Flowers.

Chemical constituents:

Roots – β-Sitosterol.

Leaves – Clerosterol, Campestrol, Cholesterol, Sitosterol, Stigmasterol.

Flower – Fumaric acid, β-Sitosterol.

Folk Use: Miscarriages

Use in literature:

Roots – Skin diseases, Tumour.

Leaves – Bronchitis, Cough, General debility, Helminthiasis, Inflammation, Intermittent fever, Leprosy, Malaria fever, Skin diseases, Tumours.

93. *Clitoria ternatea* L. (Papilionaceae)

Vern.: Visnukanta.

Distribution: On roadside bushes. Chhindwara, Hosahangabad, Indore, Jabalpur, Mandla, Raisen, Ratlam, Rewa, Sagar, Satna, Seoni, Shahdol, Shivpuri, Sidhi, W. Nimar.

Botany: Twinning herbs, with imparipinnate, 5 to 7-foliate leaves and blue or white flowers. Pods spreading.

Flowering & Fruiting: July-March

Medicinal Parts: Root.

Chemical constituents: Root bark contains Starch, Tannin, Resin.

Seeds contain Oil, bitter blue coloured resin.

Folk Use: Snake bite

Use in literature: Root – Amentia, asthma, bronchitis, burning sensation, elephantiasis, fevers, helminthiasis, inflammation, leprosy, leucoderma, Ophthalmopathy, strangury, tubercular glands, ulcers.

Leaves – Eruptions, hepatopathy, Otalgia.

Seed – Visceralgia.

94. *Coccinia cordifolia Cogn.* (Cucurbitaceae)

Syn.: *C. grandis* (L.) Voight.; *C. indica* W. & A.; *Cephalandra indica* Naud.

Vern.: Kanduri.

Distribution: Bhopal, Chhindwara, Jabalpur.

Botany: Slender, dioecious climbers; nodes on the mature stem annulate; leaves entire or digitately 3-5 lobed, cordate; flowers white, usually solitary axillary; fruits oblong-obtuse, green.

Flowering & Fruiting: July-May.

Medicinal Parts: Leaves.

Chemical constituents: Root contain β- Amyrin, Lupeol, β-sitosterol.

Fruits contain Beta-amyrin, lupeol, cucerbitacin, β- sitosterol, taraxerol, lycopene, β- carotene, crypto xanthin.

Seeds contain A fat rich in palmitic, Oleic, Linoleic acids.

Folk Use: Diabetes

Use in literature: Root – Burning sensation, vomiting.

Leaf – Dyspepsia, inflammation, jaundice, leprosy, ulcers.

Fruits – Asthma, burning sensation, bronchitis, cough, diabetes, helminthiasis, jaundice, leprosy, skin diseases.

95. *Cocculus hirsutus* (L.) Diels. (Menispermaceae)

Syn.: *Menispermum hirsutum* L.; *C. villosus* DC.

Vern.: Jamtikibel.

Distribution: Over bushes & Small trees. Common throughout the State.

Botany: Scandent, dioecious shrubs, with cordate – lanceolate or subdeltoid leaves. Male flowers minute, yellowish – green, in panicles. Fruits reddish – purple, smooth; Seeds transversely rugose.

Flowering & Fruiting: November – May.

Medicinal Parts: Leaves.

Chemical constituents: Leaves contain Trilobine & Isotrilobine.

Root contains D – Trilobine, DL – Coclaurine.

Stem contains β – Sitosterol, ginnol & mono methyl ether of Inositol.

Folk Use: Eczema, Gonorrhoea

Use in literature: Root – Bronchitis, buring sensation, cephalalgia, colic, cough, dyspepsia, flatulence, fractures, general debility, gout, hypertension, intermittent fevers, leprosy, poisonous bites, pruritus, skin diseases, spermatorrhoea, strangury, tubercular glands.

Leaves – Cough, eczema, gonorrhoea, neuralgia, ophthalmia.

96. *Coleus aromaticus* Benth. (Lamiaceae)

Syn.: *C. amboinicus* Lour.

Vern.: Patthar chur.

Distribution: Planted in Gardens.

Botany: A small perennial, hairy herb. About 1-3 ft. high with thick and fleshy aromatic leaves; flowers light purple.

Flowering & Fruiting: February-March.

Medicinal Parts: Leaves.

Chemical constituents: Leaves contain Diterpene, Methylene – quinone, couleon, cyclobuta tucin.

Root contains Naphtho Pyrone (Rocetin) and Dialdehyde, Avolatile oil carvacrol is also found.

Folk Use: Vomiting, Indigestion, Lactation, Stomachache

Use in literature: Leaf – Asthma, bronchitis, cholera, colic, cough, diarrhoea, dyspepsia, epilepsy, fever, flatulence, hiccough, otalgia, renal & vesical caliculi.

97. *Commelina benghalensis* L. (Commelinaceae)

Distribution: Abundant in moist places mostly in alluvial soil, often in wastelands. Balaghat, Damoh, Hosahangabad, Indore, Mandla, Panna, Rewa, Sidhi, Tikamgarh, W. Nimar.

Botany: Diffusely branched, deumbent herbs, with elliptic-ovate leaves. Flowers blue; spathes sessile or subsessile. Capsules 3-gonous; seeds pitted. Flowering & Fruiting: August-January.

Medicinal Parts: Whole plant.

Chemical Constituents: The flower pigment contains delphinidin diglucoside as the main constituent and P-cumaric acid and awobanol.

Medicinal Properties: Dropsy

Use in literature: Whole plant – Leprosy.

98. *Convolvulus arvensis* L. (Convolvulaceae)

Distribution: Common as weed in fields, along railway tracks & forests roads. Damoh, Indore, Raisen, Satna, Seoni, Sidhi.

Botany: Creeping or twining, perennial herbs, Leaves sagittate-hastate at base, Flowers pale pink, Flowering & Fruiting: December-February.

Medicinal Parts: Whole plant, Root.

Chemical Constituents: Roots – Cuscohygrine, Coumarins.

Aerial parts – N-alkanes, N-alkanols & Sterols.

Medicinal Properties: Purgative

Use in literature: Leaves – Boils.

99. *Convolvulus pluricaulis* Choisy. (Convolvulaceae)

Vern.: Shankpushpi.

Distribution: Common in open fields, sandy and rocky places. Chhatarpur, Gwalior, Indore, Mandla, Rewa, Seoni, Sidhi.

Botany: A prostrate or suberect, spreading, hairy, perennial herb with a woody rootstock. Leaves linear-lanceolate; hairy. Flowers white or pale-rose, solitary or in pairs, sessile or subsessile in the leaf axils. Capsule oblong-globose.

Flowering & Fruiting: December-February.

Medicinal Parts: Whole plant, root, leaves, flowers.

Chemical constituents: Plant contains Alkaloid, shankhpushpin, essential oil, methyl pentos, scamonolic acid and palmintic acid, phytosterol, ipuranol, sucrose, reducing sugars, starch and olein.

Folk Use: Brain tonic, Weakness

Use in literature: Effective on brain and heart, effective on thyroid high secretion; increases memory, positive effect on blood pressure, reduces blood pressure and tension, useful in epilepsy, insomnia & mental diseaes.

100. *Corchorus olitorius* L. (Tiliaceae)

Distribution: Balaghat, Damoh, Dhar, Gwalior, Hosahangabad, E. Nimar, Mandla, Panna, Satna, Shivpuri, Sidhi.

Botany: Annual herbs, with ovate-lanceolate leaves & yellow flowers. Capsules 5-valved, 10 ribbed, with entire beak. Flowering & Fruiting: September-January.

Medicinal Parts: Seeds.

Chemical Constituents: Fibers – Cellulose, Lignin, Nitrogen, Fat, Wax.

Seeds – Crude protein, Crude fibre, Free invert sugar, Minerals; Fixed oil; Fatty acids; Oleic & Linoleic acid, Arachidic acid, Palmitic, Stearic acid; Crystalline Substance-Corchoritin.

Folk Use: Hair fall, Stomachache

Use in literature: Leaves – Abdominal tumours, Ascites, Pain, Piles, Tumours.

101. *Cordia dichotoma* Forst. f. (Boraginaceae)

Syn.: *C. obliqua* Willd.; *C. myxa* Roxb. non L.; *C. latifolia* Roxb.

Vern.: Gunda.

Distribution: Common along roadsides, near villages and forest edges. Chhatarpur, Damoh.

Botany: Deciduous trees, with 3 to 5-nerved, elliptic-ovate or obovate leaves longer than broad. Flowers white, in dichotomous cymes. Fruits globose, yellow to red when ripe.

Flowering & Fruiting: March- July.

Medicinal Parts: Bark, leaves.

Chemical constituents: Bark contains Tannins, allantonin, B-sitosterol, a flavanone rhamnopyranoside.

Fruits contain Mucilage & sugars.

Seed oil contain B-sitosterol.

Seeds contain flavonolglycosides, taxifolin-3- rhamnoside.

Folk Use: Bodyache, Influenza

Use in literature: Bark – Burning sensation, diarrhoea, dyspepsia, fever, helminthiasis, leprosy, skin diseses.

Leaf – Gonorrhoea.

Fruits – Bronchitis, burning sensation, cough, fever, leprosy, pectoral diseases, ringworm, skin diseases, ulcers.

102. *Coriandrum sativum* L. (Apiaceae)

Vern.: Dhania.

Distribution: Widely cultivated throughout the State. Chhatarpur, Sidhi.

Botany: An annual glaberous herbs, with a strong smell; lower leaves palmatipartite, upper leaves ternately decompound; flowers white, dull purplish in the centre; fruits elliptic-orbicular, glabrous.

Flowering & Fruiting: December-April.

Medicinal Parts: Leaves, Fruits, Seed.

Chemical constituents: Leaves – Oxalic acid, calcium, vitamin-C.

Fruits – β-sitosterol, chlorogenic acid, caffic acid, umbelliferone, scopoletin.

Seeds – Quercetin 3-0-caffeyl glucoside, kaempferol 3-glucoside, fatty oil, essential oil.

Folk Use: Headache

Use in literature: Leaves – Hiccough, Inflammations, Jaundice.

Fruits – Bronchitis, burning sensation, cough, diarrhoea, dropsy, dysentery, erysipelas, helminthiasis, scrofula.

103. *Costus speciosus* (Koenig ex Retz.) J.E. Smith (Zingiberaceae)

Syn.: *Banksea speciosa* Koenig.

Vern.: Kevuk kand.

Distribution: Common in shady places along rivers or drains, sometimes in sal forests. Balaghat, Damoh, Hosahangabad, Rewa, Sidhi, W. Nimar.

Botany: An erect, herbaceous plant; leaves subsessile, arranged spirally, oblong or oblanceolate, glabrous above, thinly silky beneath; flowers white, large, many, in terminal dense heads; bracts 2-3 cm long, ovate, brownish-red or bright red; capsule subglobosely 3-gonous; seeds black with white aril.

Flowering & Fruiting: August-May.

Medicinal Parts: Rhizomes.

Chemical constituents: Rhizomes contain Alkaloids, Tigogenin, Diosgenine, Starch, β-Sterol, glucoside.

Leaves contain Alpha-Amyrin stearate, β- Amyrin and Lupeol palmitates.

Folk Use: Rheumatism, Snake bite

Use in literature: Rhizome – Anaemia, asthma, bronchitis, burning sensation, constipation, fever, flatulence, helminthiasis, hiccough, inflammation, leprosy, skin diseases.

104. *Crinum defixum* Ker.-Gwal. (Amaryllidaceae)

Vern.: Vishamandala.

Distribution: In Marshy and muddy places along streams and roadside ditches. Bhopal.

Botany: A perennial herb with avoid bulb; leaves linear, subfleshy, slightly concave, apex acute; scape 30-50 cm. long; bracts spathaceous, membranous; flowers white; fruit sub-globose, beaked; seeds 1-2, rogouse.

Flowering & Fruiting: July-October.

Medicinal Parts: Bulb.

Chemical Constituents: Bulb – Lycorine.

Folk Use: Piles.

Use in literature: Bulb – Burns, Carbuncle, Witlow.

105. *Cuminum cyminum* L. (Apiaceae)

Vern.: Jeera.

Distribution: Widely cultivated throughout the State.

Botany: Glabrous, annual herbs, with Rose-coloured flowers. Fruits setulose, narrowly oblong.

Flowering & Fruiting**:** January-March.

Medicinal Parts: Fruits.

Chemical constituents: Fruits contain Apigenin-7-O-glucoside, Luteolin-7-O-glucoside, essential oil.

Folk Use: Bad smelling of mouth

Use in literature: Fruits – Asthma, colic, dyspepsia, fever, flatulence, helminthiasis, inflammations, leprosy, leucorrhoea, skin diseases, strangury, vomiting.

106. *Curculigo orchioides* Gaertn. (Amaryllidaceae)

Syn.: *C. malabarica* Wight.; *C. brevifolia* Dryland.; *Hypoxis orchiodies* Kurz.; *Carcinia malabarica* Desv.

Vern.: Kali musli.

Distribution: In Sal forests. Throughout the State.

Botany: Perennial herbs, with thick tuberous root – stock and without aerial stem. Leaves plicate, linear – lanceolate. Flowers yellow 2 to 3 together on axillary peduncles hidden among leaf-sheaths.

Flowering & Fruiting**:** June – September.

Medicinal Parts: Root-stock.

Chemical constituents: Root stock contains Steroids–Terpenoids, Phenolics, Tannins, Glycosides, Starch, Iron, Calcium, Magnessium, Sodium, Stranthium, Resin, gum, Calcium Oxalate.

Folk Use: Asthma, Diarrhoea, Gonorrhoea, Jaundice, Piles

Use in literature: Asthma, bronchitis, colic, diarrhoea, dyspepsia, gonorrhoea, jaundice, leucorrhoea, lumbago, pruritus, skin diseases, vomiting, wounds.

107. *Curcuma amada* Roxb. (Zingiberaceae)

Vern.: Ambi haldi.

Distribution: In moist places between rock boulders or near streams. Balaghat, Bhopal, Hosahangabad, Indore, Satna, W. Nimar.

Botany: Stemless herbs, with ellipsoid, sessile tubers with the smell of unripe mango. Leaves oblong-lanceolate. Flowers white or pale – yellow, in spikes appearing with the leaves.

Flowering & Fruiting: July-October.

Medicinal Parts: Rhizomes.

Chemical constituents: Rhizome contains Essential oil (Pinene, ocimene, safrol), Resin, sugars, Gum, Starch, Albuminoids, crude fibres, organic acid, Phytosterol, zulenogeine, Camphor, curcumene, Turmerone, Volatile oil.

Folk Use: Anaemia, Sprain

Use in literature: Bronchitis, colic, constipation, cough, dyspepsia, fever, flatuance, gout, hiccough, inflammation, pruritus, skin diseases, ulcers, wounds.

108. *Curuma longa* L. (Zingiberaceae)

Syn.: *C. domestica* Valeton.; *C. rotunda* L.; *Amomum curcuma* Jacq.

Vern.: Haldi.

Distribution: Cultivated. Bhopal, Indore and other districts of the State.

Botany: Rhizomes large, yielding turmeric. Leaves oblong-elliptic. Flowers pale-yellow.

Flowering-Fruiting: September-November.

Medicinal Parts: Rhizomes.

Chemical constituents: Rhizome contains Active curcumin compound; essential oils-Termeric oil, Terpenoids, A volatile oil: it contains curcumen (Terpene), starch, Albumnoids.

Folk Use: Vomiting

Rhizome – Acrid, alterative, anodyne, anthelmintic, anti – inflammatory, antiperiodic, antiseptic, appetiser, bitter, carminative, depurative, diuretic, emollient, expectorant, febrifuge, laxative, stimulant, stomachic, thermogenic.

Use in literature: Rhizome – Amenorrhoea, anaemia, asthma, bronchitis, colic, conjunctivitis, constipation, cough, diabetes, dropsy, dyspepsia, elephantiasis, fever, flatulence, gonorrohoea, haemorrhoges, helminthiasis, hiccough, hysteria, inflammation, jaundice, leprosy, pruritus, ringworm, skin diseases, ulcers, wounds.

109. *Cuscuta reflexa* Roxb. (Convolvulaceae)

Vern.: Amarbel.

Distribution: Common on a variety of hosts. Balaghat, Betul, Chhatarpur, Damoh, Hosahangabad, Indore, Narsimhapur, Seoni, Shahdol, Sidhi.

Botany: Leafless stem – parasites, with greenish – yellow stem. Flowers whitish, solitary or in clusters arranged in racemes; style 1; stigmas 2.

Flowering & Fruiting: November-March.

Medicinal Parts: Whole plant.

Chemical constituents: Plant contains Alkaloids, proteins, flavonoids, resin, tannins, glycosides, carbohydrates, cuscutin, cuscatalin, reducing sugars.

Seeds contain Fixed oil, Amarbelin (Pigment.), bitter resin, aluminum, calcium, sodium, potassium & reducing sugars.

Folk Use: Anthelmintic, Epilepsy, Rheumatism

Use in literature: Whole plant – Bronchitis, cough, fever, Jaundice, paralysis.

110. *Cymbopogon martinii* (Roxb.) Wats. (Poaceae)

Syn.: *Andropogon martini* Roxb.

Vern.: Rosha.

Distribution: Common. Gwalior, Hosahangabad, Sidhi.

Botany. Tufed, sweet-scented perennial grass. Leaves amplexicaul at base. Panicles large, decompound; sessile spikeletes awned and lower glume have a deep median groove.

Flowering & Fruiting: September– February.

Medicinal Parts: Inflorescence.

Chemical constituents: Leaves contain Geranium oil.

Folk Use: Typhoid.

Use in literature: Bronchitis, catarrh, cardiac debility, colic, cough, dyspepsia, fever, helminthiasis, leprosy, skin diseases.

111. *Cynodon dactylon* (L.) Pers. (Poaceae)

Syn.: *Panicum dactylon* L.

Vern.: Dub.

Distribution: Common throughout the State.

Botany: Creeping, rhizomatous grass. Ligule a ring of hairs. Spikes 2-6, up to 6 cm long; lemmas longer than upper glumes, simple hairy. Grains turgid.

Flowering & Fruiting: Most throughout the year.

Medicinal Parts: Leaves, Whole plant.

Chemical constituents: Plant containsβ- Sitosterol, β- Carotene, Vitamin- C, Carotenes, Glucosides, Palmitic acid, Triterpenoid, Arundoin, Friedelene, Alkaloids – Erganovin, Erganovinine, ferulic, mono & oligo, Saccharide- glucose, fructose, sucrose, starch & lignin.

Folk Use: Bleeding, Diarrhoea, Dysentery, Epilepsy, Eye pain, Rheumatism

Use in literature: Abortion, Burning sensation, conjunctivitis, diarrhea, dysentery, general debility, haemorrhages, haemorrhoids, leprosy, skin diseases, vomiting, wounds.

112. *Cyperus rotundus* L. (Cyperaceae)

Syn.: *C. hexastachys* Rottb.

Vern.: Motha.

Distribution: In open moist places. Betul, Damoh, Hosahangabad, Indore, Mandla, Rewa, Satna, Seoni, Sidhi, Ujjain, W. Nimar.

Botany: Sedges, with slender stolons terminated by ellipsoid or globose-ovoid tubers. Leaves not exceeding the clum. Spikes born in terminal corymbs; spikelets dusty brown, 8 to 28 flowered; rachilla winged. Achenes triquetrous, brown.

Flowering & Fruiting: July-April.

Medicinal Parts: Tubers.

Chemical constituents: Rhizome contains Essential oil which contains; Penene, cineol; fatty oil which contains; Linoleic acid, oleic acid, Myristic acid, Stearic; Glycerol, Glycoside cyperene, cyperenone, sugars, gum, carbohydrates.

Leaves contain Luteolin.

Folk Use: Snake bite, Stomach disorders, Diuretic, Dyspepsia

Use in literature: Amenorrhoea, amentia, bronchitis, colic, cough, diarrhoea, dysmenorrhoea, dysentery, dyspepsia, epilepsy, fever, flatulence, general calculi, general debility, inflammation, leprosy, pruritus, scabies, skin diseases, ulcer, verminosis, vomiting, wounds.

113. *Dalbergia sissoo* Roxb. (Papilionaceae)

Vern.: Shisham.

Distribution On rosdsides and in mixed forests. Balaghat, Bhopal, Chhatarpur, Damoh, Gwalior, Hosahangabad, Indore, Jabalpur, Mandla, Ratlam, Rewa, Sagar, Satna, Seoni, Shahdol, Shivpuri, Sidhi.

Botany: Deciduous tree, with 3-5, acuminate leaflets. Flowers yellowish, in axillary panicles. Stamens 9.

Flowering & Fruiting: February-June.

Medicinal Parts: Root, Leaves, bark, heartwood.

Chemical constituents: Plant contains Dalbergin, dalbergenone, methyl dalbergin, nordalbergin, Isodalbergin, dalbergiphenol, tecterigenin, Isocaviudin, glucoside, Isocaviunin, essential oil which contain: Bisboline & nerolidol.

Folk Use: Diarrhoea, Leucorrhoea

Use in literature: Root – Diarrhoea, dysentery.

Leaf – Buring sensation, colic, diarrhoea, dysentery, dyspepsia, gonorrhoea, menorrhoea, vomiting.

Bark/heartwood – Amenorrhoea, dysmenorrhoea, burning sensation, bronchitis, dysentery, dyspepsia, fever, gout, hiccough, inflammation, leprosy, leucoderma, scabies, sciatica, skin diseases, syphilis, ulcers, vomiting.

114. *Datura metel* L. (Solanaceae)

Syn.: *D. alba* Nees.; *D. fastuosa* L. var. *alba* C. B. Clarke.

Vern.: Kala dhatura.

Distribution: In wastelands and near drains throughout the State. Bhopal, Chhatarpur, Damoh, Indore.

Botany: A shrubby herb with dichotomous branches. Leaves ovate, sinuate, unequal sided at the base. Flowers purple or white, large, funnel shaped. Persistent calyx. Capsule globose, prickled.

Flowering & Fruiting: July – March.

Medicinal Parts: Leaves, Seed.

Chemical constituents: Seeds & flowers contain Daturadiol, Daturalone, fastusine, β- sitosterol, hyosine, hyoscyamine, atropine, fastudin, fastunine, fastusic acid, fastusidine, fastusinine, daluranlone, citrostadienol, obtusifoliol, allantoin, caproic, β- linolic, linoleic acid, oteic acid, datumetine, datumetelin, vitamin- C, chlorogenic acid, fixed oil.

Folk Use: Asthma, Rheumatism, Snake bite

Use in literature: Leaf – Asthma, dandruff, epilepsy, lumbago, mumps, neuralgia, otalgia, sciatica, swellings.

Seed – Asthma, otalgia, skin diseases.

115. *Datura stramonium* L. (Solanaceae)

Syn.: *D. tatula* L.

Vern.: Safed dhatura.

Distribution: In Wastelands throughout the State.

Botany: An erect, annual herb; leaves sinuate, lanceolate, acute at apex, narrowed at base, membranous, sparsely pubescent; flowers white; capsule erect, oblong, densely covered with long prickles.

Flowering & Fruiting: November-March.

Medicinal Parts: Leaves.

Chemical constituents: Plant contains Hysocyamine, hyoscine, atropine, scopalamine, tigloidin, tropine, linoleic acid, legnoceric, myristic, palmitic acid, oleic, stearic acid, β- carbolines, compesterol, β-sitosterol, stigmasterol, β- amyrin, daturadiol, gramisterol, chlorogenic acid, datugen, datugenine, daturalactone, stramonolide.

Folk Use: Inflammation, Joints swelling, Lumbago

Use in literature: Seed – Biliousness, itching, jaundice, leucoderma, piles, skin diseases, ulcer.

116. *Desmodium gangeticum* (L.) DC. (Papilionaceae)

Syn.: *D. collinum* Roxb.; *Hedysarum gangetium* L.

Vern.: Sarivan.

Description: In Sal and Teak forests. Balaghat, Bhopal, Chhindwara, Damoh, Gwalior, Hosahangabad, Indore, Jabalpur, Mandla, Narsimhapur, Panna, Raisen, Rewa, Satna, Seoni, Shahdol, Shivpuri, Sidhi, Tikamgarh.

Botany: Undershrub; leaflets ovate-oblong; flowers purple-pink, clustered in racemes; pods linear, flat, falcate.

Flowering & Fruiting: July-April.

Medicinal Parts: Roots.

Chemical constituents: Plant contains Pterocarpanoids, Gangetin, gengetinin, Desmodin, alkaloids, Isoflavonoid, Phytoalexins, Isoflavones, genestein.

Folk Use: Asthma, Cough, Dysentery, Fever, Spermatorrhoea, Tonic

Use in literature: Root – Asthma, debility, bronchitis, cough, dysentery, dyspepsia, fever, gout, haemorrhoids, inflammation.

117. *Desmodium triflorum* (L.) DC. (Papilionaceae)

Distribution: Along sreams. Balaghat, Bhind, Bhopal, Chhindwara, Damoh, Hosahangabad, Indore, Mandla, Morena, Narsimhpur, Panna, Raisen, Rewa, Sagar, Shivpuri, Sidhi.

Botany: A much branched, gregarious, wiry, trailing herbs, rooting at the nodes. Leaflets obovate, obcordate. Flowers Pink or Purplish, 1-3 in the axils of leaves. Pods curved, flat, indented on the lower edge, 3 to 5 jointed. Seeds Brown.

Flowering & Fruiting: September-April.

Medicinal Parts: Whole plant, Leaves.

Chemical Constituents: Root / Leave / Stem – Trigonelline, Stachydrine, Betaine, Choline, Indole-3-acetic acid, Tyramine, Hypaphorin, 4β-Phenylethylamines.

Folk Use: Breast pain, Fever, Toothache

Use in literature: The plant is useful in Bronchitis, Burning sensation, Cough, Dysentery, Erysipelas, Flatulence, Pruritus, Wounds.

118. *Dichrostachys cinerea* (L.) W. & A. (Mimosaceae)

Syn.: *Mimosa cinerea* L.

Vern.: Bilatri, Sagun Kanti.

Distribution Distribution: In dry deciduous forests. Damoh, Hosahangabad, Seoni, Shahdol, Shivpuri.

Botany: Polygamous shrubs, with branches ending into spines. Pinnae 4-14 pairs and leaflets 12-24 pairs. Spikes yellow in upper half and rose-pink or purple below. Pods twisted torulose.

Flowering & Fruiting: June-January.

Medicinal Parts: Root.

Folk Use: Rheumatism

Use in literature: Diarrhoea, dyspepsia, elephantiasis, inflammation.

119. *Dioscorea bulbifera* L. (Dioscoreaceae)

Syn.: *D. versicolor* Buch. Ham.; *D. pulchella* Roxb.; *D. sativa* Thunb.; *C. crispata* Roxb.

Vern.: Varahi kand.

Distribution: Common in mixed and Sal forests. Balaghat, Sidhi.

Botany: Slender, glabrous, twining herbs with globose to pyriform tubers; leaves broadly ovate, glabrous, acuminate, with a deeply cordate base; male flowers in raceme like, axillary spikes, greenish-purple; female flowers sessile, axillary or in fascicled spikes, purple; capsule quadrately oblong.

Flowering & Fruiting: November-January.

Medicinal Parts: Tubers.

Chemical constituents: Plant contains A poisonous glucoside (Dioscorine).

Tuber contains Starch, Vitamin – B, Calcium oxalate, Protein, Iron.

Folk Use: Piles, Syphilis

Use in literature: Tuber – Biliousness, bronchitis, dyspepsia, leucoderma, piles, strangury, tumors, urinary discharges.

120. *Diospyros melanoxylon* Roxb. (Ebenaceae)

Syn.: *D. tupru* Buch.-Ham.

Vern.: Biripatta, Tendu.

Distribution: Common in dry deciduous forests and roadsides. Balaghat, Damoh, Hosahangabad, Indore, Jabalpur, Mandla, Morena, Panna, Satna, Seoni, Shivpuri, Sidhi.

Botany: Deciduous trees, with sub-opposite & alternate, ovate-elliptic leaves. Male flowers in drooping cymes; anthers awnless. Fruits globose or ovoid.

Flowering & Fruiting: March-August.

Medicinal Parts: Bark, Leaves, Unripe Fruits, Seed.

Chemical Constituents: Bark – Tannins.

Folk Use: Diarrhoea, Dysentery, Snake bite

Use in literature: Dried flowers – Urinary, Skin & Blood diseases.

Bark – Diarrhoea, Dyspepsia.

121. *Diplocyclos palmatus* (L.) Jeffrey (Cucurbitaceae)

Syn.: *Bryonia laciniosa* L.; *B. palmata* L.; *Bryonopsis laciniosa* (L.) Naud.

Vern.: Shivlingi.

Distribution: Hoshangabad, Morena, Sidhi.

Botany: Climbers, with 2-fid tendrils and 5-lobed leaves. Flowers greenish- yellow. Fruits globose, 6-striped; seeds with raised projections on both faces.

Flowering & Fruiting: December-January.

Medicinal Parts: Seed.

Chemical constituents:

Seed oil Punicic acid.

Folk Use: Promote conception

Use in literature: Cough, flatulences, general debility, inflammation, skin diseases.

122. *Drypetes roxburghii* (Wall.) Hurus. (Euphorbiaceae)

Syn.: *Putranjiva roxburghii* Wall.

Vern.: Putranjiva.

Distribution: Commonly planted as avenue tree, sometimes in wastelands Chhatarpur, Damoh, Indore, Rewa, Seoni.

Botany: Evergreen trees, with pendent branches and elliptic-oblong leaves. Flowers dioecious, apetalous, fascicled in axillary clusters. Fruits ellipsoid, hard.

Flowering & Fruiting: March –February.

Medicinal Parts: Leaf, seed.

Chemical constituents: Fruit contains Manitol, Saponins.

Seed contains Arachidic acid, Linoleic acid, Palmitic acid, Stearic acid, Glucochlearin, Glucocleomin, Gluco Putranjivin, Putranjivoside, Putranoside, β- Sitosterol.

Leaves contain Stigmasterol.

Bark contains Carboxylic acid, Putric acid, Putranjivic acid.

Folk Use: Rheumatism

Use in literature: Leaf – Catarrh, fever, sterility.

Seed – Azoospermia, burning sensation, constipation, elephantiasis, inflammation, sterility.

123. *Echinops echinatus* Roxb. (Asteraceae)

Vern.: Ontkata.

Distribution: Common in dry wasteland, ridges and boundaries of cultivated fields. In dry deciduous forests. Damoh, Shivpuri, Sidhi.

Botany: Thistle-like annual herbs, with pinnatifid, spinescent leaves white woolly beneath. Heads white, blue or yellow, 1- flowered clustered in spinos globose compound heads.

Flowering & Fruiting: October – March.

Medicinal Parts: Root.

Chemical constituents:

Plant Hentriacontane, hentriacontanol, B-amyrin and leupeol.

Seeds Echinopsine.

Folk Use: Cold, Fever, Sore throat, Vomiting

Use in literature: Biliousness, diseases of the heart, gleet, strangury, urinary discharges.

124. *Eclipta prostrata* (L.) L. (Asteraceae)

Syn.: *E. alba* Hassak.

Vern.: Bhangra.

Distribution: Common in moist waste places. Damoh.

Botany: Erect or prostate herbs, often rooting at the lower nodes. Leaves elliptic-oblong. Heads white, solitary.

Flowering & Fruiting: Throughout the year.

Medicinal Parts: Seed oil, Leaves, Whole plant.

Chemical constituents: Plant contains Glucosides – phytosterol – A, β- Amyrin, wedelolactone, luteoline, triterpenic acid, fatty acids, palmitic acid, stearic acid, oleic acid, linolic acid, nicotine, ampliptene alkaloid, ecliptine & resin.

Folk Use: Antiseptic, Asthma, Hair growth

Use in literature: Debility, elephantiasis, fever, hypertension, inflammation, jaundice, leprosy, otalgia, pruritus, skin diseases, ulcers, wounds.

125. *Emilia sonchifolia* (L.) DC. (Asteraceae)

Distribution: Common along river banks; on sandy soil. Damoh, Hosahangabad, Sidhi.

Botany: Variously branched procumbent annual herbs, with Purple flowers and Achene fruits.

Flowering & Fruiting: February-March.

Medicinal Parts: Whole plant.

Chemical Constituents: Aerial parts contain Kaempferol-3β-D Galactoside, Quercitrin, Rutin, Quercetin, Ursolic acid, N-hexacosanol, Triacontane, Hyperoside, Pyrrolizidine, Alkaloids as Senkirkine, Cloronine, β-Sitosterol, Ralmitic acid, Stigmasterol.

Folk Use: Bowel complaint, Diarrhoea, Ear sores, Night blindness

Use in literature: The plant is useful in Asthma, Cuts, Diarrohea, Intermittent Fever, Ophthalmia, Otalgia, wounds.

126. *Enicostemma littorale* Blume. (Gentianaceae)

Syn.: *E. axillare* (Lam.) Raynal.

Vern.: Nau.

Distribution: Along Ponds. Chhatarpur, Damoh.

Botany: Perennial herb, with 4-angular branches and linear-lanceolate leaves. Flowers white, in axillary clusters. Capsules 1-celled, 2-valved.

Flowering & Fruiting: July – October.

Medicinal Parts: Whole plant.

Chemical constituents: Swertiamarin, gentianine, apigenin, genkwanin, Isovitexin, saponarin, heptacosane, nonacosane, myristic acid, oleic acid, gentiocrucine, alkaloids.

Folk Use: Fever, Gout, Haeadache

Use in literature: Constipating, dyspepsia, dropsy, fever leprosy, pruritus, skin diseases, swelling.

127. *Erythrina variegata* L. (Papilionaceae)

Syn.: *E. indica* Lam.

Vern.: Paribhadra.

Distribution: Planted as an ornamental. Bhopal, Indore, Seoni.

Botany: Small tree, with 3-foliate leaves, red flowers and black, torulose pods.

Flowering & Fruiting: March-September.

Medicinal Parts: Bark.

Chemical constituents: Bark contains A bitter erytherine alkaloid & resins.

Leaves contain Erytherine, alkaloid.

Folk Use: Loose Motion, Boils, Headache.

Use in literature: Bark – Colic, conjunctivitis, cough, dyspepsia, fevers, inflammation, insomnia, leprosy, otalgia, skin diseases.

Leaf – Dysmenorrhoea, otalgia.

128. *Eulophia nuda* Lindl. (Orchidaceae)

Distribution: In Sal forests, alongwith Elephantopus scaber. Balaghat.

Botany: Terrestrial orchid; with tuberous roots & Whitish-Purple flowers in spadix inflorescence.

Flowering & Fruiting: April-September.

Medicinal parts: Tubers.

Chemical constituents:

Tuber contains – Eulophiol, n-hexacosyl alcohol, Nudol, Lupeol.

Folk Use: Blood diseases, Bronchitis, Snake bite

Use in literature:

Tuber – Intestinal worms, Tumours, Bronchitis, Diseases of the Blood.

129. *Euphorbia hirta* L. (Euphorbiaceae)

Syn.: *E. pilulifera* L.

Vern.: Dudhi.

Distribution: Common along roadsides and waste moist places. Balaghat, Chhatarpur, Damoh, Hosahangabad, Indore, Jabalpur, Satna, Tikamgarh.

Botany: Erect or procumbent herbs, with ovate-lanceolate or rhomboid-oblong leaves. Cyathia greenish, crowded in pedunculate cymes; glands stalked, pink. Capsules globosely 3-gonous.

Flowering & Fruiting**:** Throghout the year.

Medicinal Parts: Whole plant.

Chemical constituents: Plant contains Quercetin, Triacentane, ellagic acid, Phenolics, Euphosterol, Phytosterol, Phytosterolin, Gallic, mellistic, palmitic, oleic, linoleic acid, zanthorhamnin wax, chlorophyll, resin, tannins, sugar, mucilage, carbohydrates, albuminoids, catchin, oxalate.

Folk Use: Asthma, Colic pain, Dysentery, Lactaion, Urinogenital diseases

Use in literature: Asthma, colic, cough, dysentery, gonorrhoea, intestinal worms in children, leucoderma.

130. *Euphorbia neriifolia* L. (Euphorbiaceae)

Vern.: Pattonkisend.

Distribution: Usually in drier or rocky regions, wastelands and often planted as hedge around the villages and cultivated fields. Damoh, E. Nimar, Hosahangabad, Panna, Seoni, Sidhi, Tikamgarh.

Botany: Erect deciduous shrubs or small trees; stem 5-angled. Leaves obovate-oblong, crowded at the end of stem, subfleshy. Involucre 3-nate; glands without petaloid limb. Capsules obovoid-trigonous, deep red or pale brown.

Flowering & Fruiting: November-December.

Medicinal Parts: Roots, stem, leaves.

Chemical constituents: Plant contains Euphol, taraxerol, friedelan, resin, gum.

Bark contains n- Hexacosonal, Euphorbol, Hexacos

Anoate, Pelargonine, diglusoside, Euphorbin.

Root & bark contains Methylene Cycloartenol, Tulipanin 3-5 diglucoside.

Folk Use: Cough, Rheumatism, Sore throat

Use in literature: Plant – Abdominal trouble, anaemia, bronchitis, fever, inflammation, leucoderma, piles, tumours, ulcer.

Milk – Abdominal pain, leucoderma, tumor.

Leaf – Abdominal trouble, inflammation, swelling, tumour.

131. *Euphorbia nivulia* Buch-Ham. (Euphorbiaceae)

Vern.: Katathohar.

Distribution: Common on slopes & foot hills. Chhatarpur, Damoh, Mandla, Rewa, Satna, Seoni.

Botany – Tall shrubs or small trees with whorled cylindrical fleshy stems and branches, covered with pairs of straight spines, leaves 15 cm. or more long.

Flowering & Fruiting: March-May.

Medicinal parts – Leaves.

Chemical constituents:

Stem – Taraxerol, Sitosterol.

Root bark – Euphol, Euphorbol, Hexacozoate.

Latex – Cyclolaudenol, Cyclonivuliaol, Cycloartenol, Cycloeucalenol.

Folk Use: Earache

Use in literature:

Latex – Asthma, Bitter, Diuretic, Digestive, Earache, Flatulence, Intermittent fever, Jaundice, Leprosy, Rheumatism, Scabies, Warts, Ulcers.

132. *Euphorbia thymifolia* L. (Euphorbiaceae)

Distribution: Common in moist places and along the roads and ridges. Balaghat, Damoh, E. Nimar, Indore, Mandla, Panna, Rewa, Sagar.

Botany: An annual herb. Leaves very small and opposite. Involucers axillary, solitary or 2-3 in an axil. Capsules erect, obtusely keeled; styles short, 2-fid. Flowering & Fruiting**:** Throughout the year.

Medicinal Parts: Whole plant.

Chemical Constituents: Plant contains Epitaraxerol, N-hexacosanol, Euphorbol, Esters, N-alkanes, Sterols, Corilagin, Geraniin, Bixanin, Casuarin, Desgalloylstachyurin.

Folk Use: Dysentery, Small pox

Use in literature: Amenorrhoea, Asthma, Bronchitis, Bleeding, Piles, Cardiac debility, Chronic Cough, Dandruff, Dysentery, Dysmenorrhoea, Flatulence, Gonorrhoea, Helminthiasis, Leprosy, Skin diseases, Strangury, Wounds.

133. *Euphorbia tirucalli* L. (Euphorbiaceae)

Vern.: Thor.

Distribution: Rare. In drier places of hilly or rocky regions. Chhatarpur, Damoh, Indore, Tikamgarh.

Botany: Shrubs or small trees, with smooth, spreading, terete, rush-like, almost leafless branches.

Flowering & Fruiting**:** August– September.

Medicinal Parts: Latex.

Chemical constituents: Stem & latex contain β- Sterol, Taraxerol.

Bark & root contain Euphorbol, Hexacosanoate, Taraxerone, Ingenol, Triacetate, Euphorginol.

Stem containEllagic acid, Kaempferol, compesterol, Stigma – Sterol.

Latex contain Amyrin, Euphol, Euphorbinol, Tirucallol, Palmitic acid.

Folk Use: Rheumatism

Use in literature: Plant – Biliousness, leprosy, leucorrhoea.

Milk – Abdominal trouble, tumour.

134. *Evolvulus alsinoides* L. (Convolvulaceae)

Syn.: *E. hirsutus* Lamk.

Vern.: Nil Shankhpuspi.

Distribution: Common in wastelands and dry mixed deciduous forests, mostly in rockey and dry places. Balaghat, Chhatarpur, Damoh, Indore, Rewa, Satna, Seoni, Shivpuri, Sidhi, W. Nimar.

Botany: Prostrate or ascending herbs, with lanceolate-oblong leaves. Flowers pale-blue, on 1 to few flowered filiform peduncles. Calyx-lobes acute. Capsules 4-valved, 4-seeded.

Flowering & Fruiting: July – March.

Medicinal Parts: Leaves.

Chemical constituents: Plant contains Yellow fatty elements, Minerals, Organic acid & Saline.

Folk Use: Asthma, Increase memory, Insomnia

Use in literature: Plant – Biliousness, bronchitis, epilepsy, leucoderma, teething in infants.

135. *Ficus benghalensis* L. (Moraceae)

Vern.: Bargad.

Distribution: Common throughout the State on roadsides, in rural areas and secondary forests. Chhatarpur, Damoh, Hosahangabad, Indore, Panna, Rewa, Sagar, Satna, Seoni, Sidhi, Tikamgarh, W. Nimar.

Botany: Large, evergreen trees, with prop roots and ovate-oblong leaves. Receptacles geminate, axillary, globose, red when ripe.

Flowering & Fruiting: August – July.

Medicinal Parts: Latex.

Chemical constituents: Plant contains Glucoside; Bengalenoside & Talbutamide; Leucoanthocyanidins, Phytosterolin, β- sitosterol, freidelin, quercetin, Galactoside, ticlic acid, tannin.

Folk Use: Diarrhoea, Dysentery, Rheumatism

Use in literature: Biliousness, erysipelas, fever, inflammation, ulcers, vaginal complaint, vomiting.

136. *Ficus glomerata* Roxb. (Moraceae)

Syn.: *F. racemosa* L.

Vern.: Gular.

Distribution: In wastelands and mixed forests, on the bank of drains and rivers. Balaghat, Chhatarpur, Damoh, Dhar, Hosahangabad, Jabalpur, Jhabua, Mandla, Panna, Rewa, Sagar, Satna, Seoni, Shivpuri, Sidhi, W. Nimar.

Botany: A large tree; leaves alternate, ovate, elliptic-lanceolate, or ovate-oblong, glabrous. Receptacles 2-4 cm across, clustered on short leafless branchlets, globose or pyriform, hairy, supported by 3 bracts at the base, green, turning reddish-purple when ripe.

Flowering & Fruiting: February – June.

Medicinal Parts: Whole plant, roots, leaves, bark, fruits, latex.

Chemical constituents: Bark contains Cerylbehenate, Lupeol, Alphaamyrin, Glaunol, β- sitosterol, keton, Hentriacontane, tiglic acid, glucose, Taraxeroll & Tannin.

Folk Use: Diabetes, Dysentery, Fever, Gonorrhoea, Piles

Use in literature: Root – Hydrophobia.

Fruits – Biliousness, blood diseases, burning sensation, fatigue, leprosy, menorrhagia, nose bleeding, urinary discharges.

137. *Ficus religiosa* L. (Moraceae)

Vern.: Pipal.

Distribution: Common throughout the State on road sides, bank of drains and rivers, in fields, villages and sometimes in forests. Balaghat, Bhopal, Chhatarpur, Damoh, Indore, Jabalpur, Panna, Shivpuri, Sidhi, W. Nimar.

Botany: Large, deciduous trees, with ovate to ovate-suborbicular leaves caudate-acuminate at apex and rounded at the base. Receptacles in axillary pairs, reddish-purple when ripe.

Flowering & Fruiting: April –September.

Medicinal Parts: Leaves.

Chemical constituents: Bark contains Tannin.

Folk Use: Snake bite

Use in literature: Burning sensation, biliousness, diseases of the blood, uterus, vagina; leucorrhoea, ulcers.

Fruits – Biliousness, burning sensation, diseases of the blood & heart.

Root – gout

Root bark – Leucorrhoea, stomatitis, ulcers.

Seed – Urinary discharges.

138. *Flacourtia indica* (Burm. f.) Merr. (Flacourtiaceae)

Syn.: *F. ramantchi* L. Herit.; *F. ramontchi* L. Herit.; *F. intermis* auct. (non Roxb.); *F. latifolia* Cooke; *F. occidentalis* Blatter; *F. cataphracta.*; *F. sapida* Roxb.; *F. sepiaria* Roxb.

Vern.: Bilanga.

Distribution: In scrub forests. In almost all the Districts.

Botany: Deciduous thorny trees, with ovate-elliptic or suborbicular leaves and greenish-yellow flowers.

Flowering & Fruiting: March-May.

Medicinal Parts: Root, Leaves, Stem Bark, Fruits.

Chemical constituents: Bark contains Tannin & flacourtin (A Phenolic glucoside ester).

Folk Use:Conjunctivitis, Leucorrhoea, Liver problem, Menstrual disorders, Rheumatism

Use in literature: Roots – Erysipelas, poisonous bites, pruritus, skin diseases, strangury.

Leaves – Pruritus, scabies.

Fruits – Jaundice, strangury.

139. *Foeniculum vulgare* Mill. (Apiaceae)

Vern.: Saunf.

Syn.: *F. capillaceus* Gilb.; *Anethum foeniculum* L.; *A. officinale* All.

Distribution: Often cultivated for fruits which are used as spices.

Botany: A large annual herb, pinnately compound leaves; Flowers yellow in compound umbels; cremocarp of 2 carples or mericarp, each one in 5-ridged furrowed. Flowering & Fruiting: December-March.

Medicinal Parts: Fruits.

Chemical constituents: Constituents of plant are Fatty oil, protein, anethose, fenchone, anisalehyde, feniculin, nelumboside; Flavons, abscisic acid. Essential oil from fruit anethole, xanthotoxin, bergapten, psoralen, scoparone, vanillin, α-pinene, camphene, limonene, α-phellandrene, fenchone, methylchavicol.

Folk Use: Kidney stone, Vomiting

Use in literature: Fruits – Anaemia, bruning sensation, bronchitis, cardiac diseases, colic, cough, dysentery, dyspepsia, dysuria, fever, flatulence, inflammation, skin diseases, vomiting.

140. *Fumaria indica* (Hassk.) Pugsley (Fumariaceae)

Syn.: *F. vaillantii* Loisel.; *F. parviflora* Lam.

Vern.: Pitpapra.

Distribution: A weed in cultivated fields. Chhatarpur, damoh, satna, shahdol.

Botany: Annual herbs; leaves 2-3 pinnatisect, segments linear-oblanceolate; flowers purplish-red, spurred, in terminal or leaf opposed, bracteate racemes; sepals inciso-dentate; nuts subglobose, rugose when dry.

Flowering & Fruiting: January – April.

Medicinal Parts: Whole plant.

Chemical constituents: Plant contains Fumaric acid & fumarin alkaloid.

Folk Use: Malaria fever, Pyrexia

Use in literature: Blood diseases, fever, leprosy, rhinitis, tuberculousis, vertigo.

141. *Gardenia gummifera* L. f. (Rubiaceae)

Vern.: Chhote kurra.

Syn.: *G. lucida* Roxb.

Distribution: Balaghat, Seoni.

Botany: A small compact tree; leaves simple smooth & bright; flowers white during early period but yellow later on; 1-3 in cluster, gum is secreted from tender branches and buds during winter.

Flowering & Fruiting: March-August.

Medicinal Parts: Gum.

Chemical constituents: Oleanonic aldehyde, sitosterol, D-mannitol, erythrodiol, 5-flavons, gardenin, de-me-tangeretin nevadensin.

Fruits contain Nonacosane, β-sitosterol, d-mannitol.

Folk Use: Diarrhoea, Ulcer

Use in literature: Resin – Bronchitis, cardiac debility, colic, constipation, cough, dyspepsia, fever, flatulence, hiccough, intestinal worms, leprosy, skin diseases, wounds

142. *Glinus oppositifolius* DC. (Molluginaceae)

Syn.: *Molluga oppositifolia* L.; *M. spergula* L.

Distribution: Balaghat, Damoh, Mandla, Sidhi.

Botany – Prostrate or diffuse herbs with small axillary White flowers & 3 valved capsule fruits. Flowering & Fruiting: Throughout the year.

Medicinal parts – Whole plant

Chemical constituents: Vitex, Spergulagenic acid, Oleanolic acid, Methyl Spergulagenate, Spergulagenin A.

Folk Use: Earache, Itching

Use in literature: Burning sensation, Bronchitis, Cough, Diabetes, Earache, Piles, Skin diseases.

143. *Gloriosa superba* L. (Liliaceae)

Syn.: *Methonia superba* Lamk.

Vern.: Kalihari.

Distribution: Abundant on bushes in open forests. Balaghat, Damoh, Dhar, Hosahangabad, Indore, Mandla, Satna, Seoni, Sidhi, Tikamgarh.

Botany: Climbing herbs, with alternate, opposite or whorled leaves ending in a tendril. Flowers yellow, tinged with red in upper half; tepals undulating on the margins, Capsules oblong.

Flowering & Fruiting: June-November.

Medicinal Parts: Rhizome, root.

Chemical constituents: Rhizome tubers contain Alkaloid colchicine; superbine, glorisine; sitosterol, glucosides, benzoic acid & resins.

Folk Use: Gonorrhoea, Gout, Leprosy, Rheumatism, Scorpion sting, Snake bite

Use in literature: Tuber – Abdominal pain, infalammation, itching, leprosy, piles, ulcer.

144. *Gmelina arborea* Roxb. (Verbenaceae)

Syn.: *G. rheedii* Hook.

Vern.: Kamhar.

Distribution: In sal forests. Chhatarpur, Damoh, Hosahangabad, Indore, Mandla, Seoni, Shahdol, Shivpuri.

Botany: Unarmed deciduous trees, with broadly ovate-acuminate leaves. Flowers yellow or brownish-yellow. Drupes obovoid, yellowish orange when ripe.

Flowering & Fruiting: March-June.

Medicinal Parts: Whole plant, roots, leaves, fruits.

Chemical constituents: Plant contains Lignan gmelinol & Arboreol.

Leaves contains Luteolin, Apigenin, Quercetin, β- Sitosterol, Isoarboreal, Oleic acid, Gmelanon, Gummadiol, Palmitic acid, oleic acid,Linoleic acid, Glucose, Xylose, Mannose, Arabinose, Galactose, Rhamnose, Stigmasterol, Sitgmastanol, Compestrol, Butulinol.

Folk Use: Fever, Gout, Worms

Use in literature: Root – Abdominal pain, burning sensation, fever, hallucinations, piles, urinary discharges.

Flower – Blood diseases, leprosy.

Fruits – Anaemia, leprosy, strangury, ulcers, vaginal discharges.

145. *Grewia subinaequalis* DC. (Tiliaceae)

Syn.: *G. hainesiana* Hole.

Vern.: Phalsa.

Distribution: Occasional in Sal forest. Balaghat, Hosahangabad, Satna.

Botany: Shrubs or small trees, with ovate to orbicular leaves and yellow flowers in extra-axillary cymes. Petals half the length of basal glands. Nuts 1-celled.

Flowering & Fruiting: November – May.

Medicinal Parts: Stem bark.

Chemical constituents: Plant contains Lupeol, Lupenon, Betulin, Friedelin, Taraxasterol, Beta-Amyrine, Grewionol, Kampferol, Amino acids, Citric acid, Vitamin-C.

Folk Use: Rheumatism

Use in literature: Fruits – Blood disorders, fever, heart disorders, inflammation, oedema, stomachahe.

146. *Gymnema sylvestre* (Retz.) R. Br. ex Sch. (Asclepiadaceae)

Syn.: *Asclepias geminata* Roxb.; *Periploca sylvestris* Retz.

Vern.: Gurmar.

Distribution: In sal and mixed deciduous forests. Betul, Chhatarpur, Damoh, Hosahangabad, Jabalpur, Narsimhapur, Panna, Raisen, Rewa, Satna, Shahdol.

Botany: Much branched, twining shrubs. Leaves ovate-elliptic or oblong. Cymes greenish–yellow. Follicles solitary, straight, lanceolate, tapering.

Flowering & Fruiting: October-February.

Medicinal Parts: Whole plant.

Chemical constituents: Leaves contains Gymnemic acid, quercitol, anthraquinon, saponin, calcium oxalate.

Folk Use: Diabetes, Menstrual disorders

Use in literature: Plant – Asthma, biliousness, bronchitis, burning sensation, eye complaint, heart diseases, inflammation, leucoderma, ulcer.

Fruits – Bronchitis, heart diseases, ulcers, urinary discharges.

147. *Haldina cordifolia* (Roxb.) Ridsd. (. (Rubiaceae)

Syn.: *Adina cordifolia* (Roxb.) Hook. f. ex Bran

Vern.: Haldu

Distribution: Balaghat, Betul, Chhatarpur, Damoh, Gwalior, Indore, Mandla, Panna, Satna, Seoni, Shahdol, Sidhi.

Botany: Large tree with spreading branches; leaves elliptic-oblong; flowers sweet scented; fruits fleshy.

Flowering & Fruiting: August-June.

Medicinal Parts: Stem bark.

Chemical constituents: Fruit contains Flavonoids.

Leaves contain Ursolic acid, quercetin 3–O– galactoside.

Heartwood contains Adinin pigment, tannins.

Stem bark contains Alkaloids, tannins pentosan, lignins, starch.

Root bark contains Coumarin glycoside adicardin.

Folk Use: Miscarriage, Rheumatism

Use in literature: Root – Dysentery.

Bark – Diseases of blood, inflammation, skin diseases.

148. *Hedychium coronarium* Koen. (Zingiberaceae)

Distribution: In moist places. Seoni.

Botany: Herbaceous, rhizomatous robust plants, with White or Yellow flowers & capsule fruits.

Flowering & Fruiting: August-February.

Medicinal parts: Rhizomes, Flowers.

Chemical constituents:

Rhizomes – Furanoditerpene as hedychenone.

Essential oil – β-Pinene, Limonene, β-Phellandrene, β-Caryophyllene.

Folk Use: Conjuncrivitis, Eye troubles

Use in literature:

Rhizomes – Intestinal worms, Fever, Rheumatism, Tonic.

149. *Helicteres isora* L. (Sterculiaceae)

Vern.: Marod phali.

Distribution: Common in deciduous forests and open areas. Balaghat, Damoh, Hosahangabad, Indore, Narsimhapur, Panna, Sagar, Seoni, Tikamgarh.

Botany: Shrubs, with ovate to orbicular leaves and red flowers. Fruits cylindric, woody, beaked, with spirally coiled follicles.

Flowering & Fruiting: August-June.

Medicinal Parts: Root, Leaf, Stem bark, seed, fruit.

Folk Use: Colic, Constipation, Flatulence in children, Gripping, Snake bite

Use in literature: Diarrhoea, dysentery, scabies, stomach affections.

150. *Heliotropium indicum* L. (Boraginaceae)

Vern.: Hathisunda.

Distribution: In moist wastelands. Balaghat, Damoh, Mandla.

Botany: Erect herbs, pale-violet flowers and fruit of 1-seeded nutlets. Flowering & Fruiting: Throughout the year.

Medicinal Parts: Whole plant.

Chemical Constituents: Aerial parts of the plant contains as Indicine, Echinatine, Supinine, Heleurine, Heliotrine, Lasiocarpine, Supinidine, Retranecine, Lindelofidine, Indicine-N-oxide, Indicinine,

Supinene, Rapanone, Lupeol, N-hexacosanol, Sitosterol, Stigmasterol, Campesterol, Cholinasterol.

Folk Use: Cough, Fever, Inflammation

Use in literature: Plant – Wounds, Skin affections, Rheumatism, Ulcers.

Root – Cough, Bornchitis, Fever, Ringworm, Rheumatism.

Leaves – Fever, Urticaria, Ulcers, Wounds, Gonorrhoea, Ringworm, Rheumatism, Erysipelas.

151. *Hemidesmus indicus* (L.) R. Br. (Asclepiadaceae)

Syn.: *Asclepias pseudosarsa* var. *latifolia* Roxb.; *Periploca indica* Willd.; *P. emetica* Retz

Vern.: Anantmul.

Distribution: On forest floor and twiner on a number of Plants. Betul, Chhatarpur, Hosahangabad, Panna, Seoni, Sidhi.

Botany: Glabrous, scandent undershrubs, with elliptic-oblong to linear-lanceolate leaves. Flowers dull yellow with purple eye. Follicles tapering to a point. Slightly falcate.

Flowering & Fruiting: August-January.

Medicinal Parts: Leaves, Root.

Chemical constituents: Root contains Essential oil, saponin, hemidester, hemidesmol, β- sitosterol, lupeol, tetracyclictriserpene, alcohol, resin, vasa acid, tannins.

Folk Use: Cough, Diarrhoea, Eczema, Rheumatism, Snake bite

Use in literature: Root – Asthma, diarrhoea, blood diseases, burning sensation, bronchitis, dysentery, fever, itching, leprosy, leucoderma, leucorrhoea, loss of appetite, piles, skin diseases.

152. *Hibiscus rosa-sinensis* L. (Malvaceae)

Vern.: Gurhal.

Distribution: Commonly grown in the gardens throughout Madhya Pradesh, mostly as a hedge and as an ornamental.

Botany: Evergreen shrubs, with pink, red or rosy flowers.

Flowering & Fruiting: Throughout the year.

Medicinal Parts: Flowers.

Chemical constituents: Leaves contain Alkaloids, Glycosides, Reducing sugars, Sterols, Resins, Beta-sitosterol.

Root contain Mucilage, fibres.

Flowers contain Fat, calcium, phosphorous, Thiamine, riboflavin, ascorbic acid, cyanin chloride.

Folk Use: Cough, Kidney trouble, Urinary problem

Use in literature: Cough, fever, anti-inflammatery, anti-bacterial, anti-fungal, antispasmodic, anti-viral, gonorrhoea, leucorrhoea.

153. *Holarrhena pubescens* (Buch.-Ham.) Wall. ex G. Don. (Apocynaceae)

Syn.: *H. antidysenterica* (Roxb. ex f.) Wall.; *Wrightia antidysenterica* J.Grah.; *Echites antidysenterica* Heyne.

Vern.: Kurchi.

Distribution: Common in sal and mixed deciduous forests. Balaghat, Chhatarpur, Damoh, E. Nimar, Gwalior, Hosahangabad, Indore, Jabalpur, Narsimhapur, Panna, Rewa, Satna, Seoni, Shivpuri, Sidhi.

Botany: Small trees, leaves ovate to elliptic. Flowers white, in terminal corymbose cymes, calyx lobes oblong-lanceolate, cilliate, corolla puberulous, follicles cylindric, often dotted with white spots.

Flowering & Fruiting: February – June.

Medicinal Parts: Root, stem bark, seeds..

Chemical constituents: Root bark contains Holacetine, connesine alkaloids.

Seed contains Essential oil, conessine & kurchicine alkaloids.

Stem bark contains Connesine, Holarrhenine, Holarrhimine, kurchine, kurchicine, conamine, & conimine.

Folk Use: Diarrhoea, Dysentery

Use in literature: Bark – Biliousness, diarrhoea, diseases of spleen, dysentery, fever, leprosy, piles, skin diseases.

Flower – Biliousness, blood diseases, diarrhoea, leucoderma.

Seed – Biliousness, burning sensation, dysentery, erysipelas, hallucinations, leprosy, piles, skin diseases.

154. *Holoptelea integrifolia* (Roxb.) Planch. (Ulmaceae)

Vern.: Chilbil.

Distribution: Common on roadsides and around villages. Chhatarpur, Damoh, Indore, Mandla, Sagar, Satna, Seoni, Shivpuri, Sidhi.

Botany: Large trees, with ovate, pinnately veined leaves and greenish-yellow flowers. Fruits brodly oblong to suborbicular, winged, flat, notched at apex.

Flowering & Fruiting: January-April.

Medicinal Parts: Bark, Leaves.

Folk Use: Rheumatism, Ringworm

Use in literature: Colic, diabetes, dyspepsia, flatulence, helminthiasis, inflammation, leprosy, rheumatism, skin diseases, vomiting.

155. *Homonoia riparia* Lour. (Euphorbiaceae)

Vern.: Surra.

Distribution: Common along the bank of drains & on river beds. Balaghat, Hosahangabad, W. Nimar.

Botany: Deciduous shrubs, with spikes inflorescens and capsule fruits. Flowering & Fruiting: January-April.

Medicinal Parts: Stem.

Chemical Constituents: Root contains – Fatty acids like myristic acid, Palmitic acid, Stearic acid, Oleic acid.

Leaves contain Quercetain-3-O-β-D-Glucopyranosyl (1→6) – Alpha-L-Rhamnoside, Gallic acid, Taraxerone.

Folk Use: Dandruff, Gonorrhoea, Malaria, Piles, Syphilis

Use in literature: Roots – Haemorrhoids, Vesical Calculi, Strangury, Gonorrhoea, Urethrorrhea, Syphilis.

Leaves / Fruits – Ulcers, Wounds, Skin diseases.

156. *Hybanthus enneaspermus* F. Muell. (Violaceae)

Syn.: *Viola enneasperma* L.; *V. suffruticosa* L.; *Lonidium suffruticosum* Ging.

Vern.: Ratanpurus.

Distribution: Among grasses along roadsides, forest fringes, bank of streams, amongst forest undergrowth, & in cultivated fields.

Botany: Perennial diffuse herbs; flowers Violet; Blue or Orange Red. Flowering & Fruiting: August-February.

Medicinal parts: Whole plant, Root.

Chemical constituents: Dipeptide alkaloids as Aurantimide acetate, Triterpenes as Isoarborinol & β-Sitosterol.

Folk Use: Urinary trouble

Use in literature:

Root – Gonorrhoea, Urinary problems.

Fruits – Antidote for Scorpion sting.

157. *Hygrophila auriculata* (Sch.) Heine (Acanthaceae)

Syn.: *Astercantha longifolia* Nees.

Vern.: Talmakhana.

Distribution: Common along ponds and ditches. Balaghat, Bhopal, Chhatarpur, Dhar, E. Nimar, Hosahangabad, Indore, Jabalpur, Mandla, Narsimhapur, Panna, Rewa, Sagar, Satna, Seoni, Shivpuri, Sidhi, Tikamgarh, W. Nimar.

Botany: Hispid annuals, with thickened nodes. Leaves oblong or lanceolate, in verticils of 6 at a node. Axillary spines yellow. Flowers purple-blue, in axillary whorls. Capsules linear- oblong.

Flowering & Fruiting: September-June.

Medicinal Parts: Roots, leaves, seeds.

Chemical constituents: Seed contains Yellow coloured oil; diastase, lipase, protease, salts of potassium, mucilage.

Folk Use: Jaundice, Rheumatism, Tonic

Use in literature: Latex – Abdominal trouble, anaemia, biliousness, constipation, diarrohoea, diseases of the eye, dysentery, inflammation, urinary calculi, urinary discharges.

Seed – Biliousness, blood diseases.

158. *Hyptis suaveolens* Poit. (Lamiaceae)

Vern.: Dona.

Distribution: Common as weed in Wastelands, along bank of drains, roadsides, in forest clearings, on hill slopes & among boulders. Chhatarpur, Damoh, Hosahangabad, Mandla, Rewa, Sidhi.

Botany – Herbs; flowers small, Blue, fruits Black nutlets. Flowering & Fruiting: Throughout the year.

Medicinal parts – Leaves.

Chemical constituents: Lupeol, Friedelin, Threonine, Valine, Arginine, etc. Amino acids, Essential oil, Campesterol, α-Pinene, Myrcene, β-Caryophyllene.

Folk Use: Pneumonia

Use in literature: Cough, Corryza, Skin diseases, Epistaxsis.

Leaf juice – Colic, Stomachache

159. *Impatiens balsamina* L. (Balsaminaceae)

Distribution: Balaghat, Damoh, Hosahangabad, Indore, Mandla, Panna, Rewa, Satna.

Botany – Annual herbs, with White or Pink flowers & capsule fruits. Flowering & Fruiting: July-October.

Medicinal parts: Flower.

Chemical constituents:

Seed contains – β-Sitosterol, β-amyrin, α-Spinasterol, Glucoside, Linoleic acid, Palmitic acid, Oleic acid, Arachidic acid.

Folk Use: Lumbago

Use in literature: The plant is Amenorrhoea, Urinary disorders, Rheumatism, Vomiting.

160. *Indigofera tinctoria* L. (Papilionaceae)

Vern.: Neel.

Distribution: On hill slopes and moist wasteland. Chhindwara, Damoh, Hosahangabad, Indore, Panna, Raisen, Ratlam, Sagar, Satna, Seoni, Shivpuri, Sidhi, Tikamgarh, W. Nimar.

Botany: Grey-pubescent undershrubs, with 7-13, obovate or oblanceolate leaflets. Racemes shorter than leaves. Pods deflexed, 8 to 10 seeded.

Flowering & Fruiting: July-May.

Medicinal Parts: Leaves.

Chemical constituents: Inorganic salts of Nitrogen, phosphoric acid, lime, potash, apigenin, kaempferol, luteolin, quercetin.

Seeds contain Galactomannan, galactose & mannose.

Folk Use: Eye diseases, Liver diseases, Nervous disorders

Use in literature: Root, Stem & Leaves – Asthma, bronchitis, skin diseases, ulcers.]

161. *Ipomoea carnea* Jacq. Sub spp *fistulosa* L.

(Convolvulaceae)

Vern.: Beharam

Distribution: Throughout the State.

Botany: Erect, ascending or seandent perennial undershrubs, with milky juice; stems fistular; leaves ovate-triangular with a cordate base; flowers purple in many flowered cymes; capsule globose, glabrous; seeds black, villous.

Flowering & Fruiting: Throughout the year.

Medicinal Parts: Leaves

Chemical constituents: Leaves- Ipomose, an anthracene glucoside, gum, jalapin, saponins.

Folk Use: Boils, Sprain, Swelling of joints, Wound

162. *Jasminum auriculatum* Vahl. (Oliaceae)

Vern.: Juhi.

Distribution: Near streams and also cultivated. Rewa.

Botany: A bushy or climbing shrub. Leaves with a pair of minute leaflets or simple. Flowers White, Star shaped.

Flowering & Fruiting: July-August.

Medicinal Parts: Leaves.

Chemical Constituents: Indole, Benzyl benzoate, Methyl Anthranilate, Benzyl Alcohol.

Folk Use: Oral ulcer

Use in literature: Root – Skin disease.

Flowers – Burning sensation, Hyperdipsia, Ophthalmopathy, Strangury, Ulcers.

163. *Jasminum multiflorum* (Burm. f.) Andr. (Oleaceae)

Syn.: J. pubescens Willd.; J. hirsutum Willd.

Vern.: Safed Chameli.

Distribution: Common along roadsides and often cultivated in gardens. Balaghat, Bhopal, Jabalpur, Sidhi.

Botany: A scandent or diffuse, densely pubescent shrub. Leaves simple, ovate thick, cordate. Flowers White slightly scented in terminal, many-flowered umbles. Calyx teeth 1 cm. or more in length. Flowering & Fruiting: December-June.

Medicinal Parts: Root.

Chemical Constituents: Leaves – Friedelin, Lupeol, Betulin, Alpha-amyrin, Betulinic acid, Ursolic acid, Oelanolic acid, Jasmolactones, A,B,C & D, Multiforoside, Multiroside, Jasmutiside, Multiflorin.

Folk Use: Snake bite

Use in literature: Flowers – Cephalagia, Inflammation, Rheumatism.

164. *Jasminm sambac* (Linn.) Ait. (Oleaceae)

Vern.: Mogra.

Distribution: As forest undergrowth and commonly planted in gardesn. Hosahangabad.

Botany: Scandent or climbing shrubs, with simple leaves and white flowers.

Flowering & Fruiting: April-October.

Medicinal Parts: Leaves.

Chemical constituents: Flowers contain Pyridine, nicotinate derivatives.

Folk Use: Boils

Use in literature: Leaves – Fever, skin diseases, ulcers.

Flowers – Fever, leprosy, hiccough, insanity, pruritus, ulcers, vomiting.

165. *Jatropha curcas* L. (Euphorbiaceae)

Vern.: Ratanjot.

Distribution: Common along cultivated fields and in wastelands. Balaghat, Chhatarpur, Indore, Mandla, Panna, Seoni, Shahdol, Sidhi, W. Nimar.

Botany: Eglandular, soft wooded shrubs or small trees, with 3 to 5-angled ovate-cordet leaves. Flowers greenish-yellow, in corymbose cymes. Capsules globose-ovoid.

Flowering & Fruiting: August-January.

Medicinal Parts: Root bark, leaves, stem, seeds, and latex.

Chemical constituents: Seed contains Amino acids, arachid acid, lionleic acid, myrstic acid, oleic acid, stearic acid, arabinose, glucose, rhamnose, galactose, xylose, galactouronic acid, β- sitoserol.

Stem bark contains B- Sitosterol, taraxerol.

Leaves contain Sucrose, vitexin, compesterol, triacontanol.

Folk Use: Piles, Rheumatism, Toothache

Use in literature: Fruit & seed – Abdominal complaint, anemia, biliousness, diseases of the heart, dysentery, fistula, urinary discharges.

Latex – Styptic

Root bark – Anaemia, biliousness, cough, dysentery, fistula, gum trouble, inflammation, rheumatism, swelling, tuberculosis, ulcer.

166. *Jatropha gossypifolia* L. (Euphorbiaceae)

Vern.: Lal – erenda.

Distribution: Common along roadsides and cultivated fields. Bhind, Chhatarpur, Damoh, Dhar, Mandla, Panna, Rewa, Satna.

Botany: Tall, erect, glandular hairy shrubs, with deep reddish-purple branches. Leaves orbicular to obovate. Palmately 3 to 5 lobed. Flowers blood-red. Capsules 3-lobed With oblong, strophiolate seeds.

Flowering & Fruiting: April-September.

Medicinal Parts: Bark, leaves, stem, Latex

Chemical constituents: Seed contains Alanine, arginine, cystine, glycine, leucine, methionine, valline, linoleic acid, oleic acid, palitic acid.

Leaves contain Apigenin, vitexin, Isovitexin.

Bark contain Ceryl & myricyl alcohol, palmitone, β-sitosterol.

Root contain Jatrophalones A & B.

Plant contain Gossypibetelene.

Folk Use: Bleeding Gums, Eczema, Headache, Itches

Use in literature: Leaves – Carbuncles, eczema, Itching.

Latex & seed oil – Ulcer (Externally applied).

167. *Justicia procumbens* L. (Acanthaceae)

Syn.: *Rostellularia procumbens* (L.) Nees.

Distribution: Common on rocky hill slopes. Balaghat, Hosahangabad, Indore.

Botany: A procumbent, diffuse, slender, branching annual. Flowering & Fruiting: September-December.

Medicinal parts – All parts

Chemical constituents:

Leaves contain – An essential oil which is Antifungal; Justicidins A & B (major), Diphyllin and Lignan Neojusticin.

Folk Use: Rheumatism

Use in literature: Asthma, Cough, Backache, Flatulence, Lumbago.

168. *Kalanchoe pinnata* (Lam.) Pers. (Crassulaceae)

Vern.: Pattharchur.

Distribution: Planted and found as escape on border of forests. Balaghat, Chhatarpur, Mandla.

Botany: A perennial glabrous succulent herb. Leaves opposite-decussate, Compound, Leaflets ovate or elliptic, crenate or serrate. Flowers in large spreading panicles, pendent, pale-greenish and reddish-purple.

Flowering & Fruiting: October-February.

Medicinal Parts: Leaves and Its juice.

Chemical constituents: Leaves contain Alkanes, Tricontane, Alpha- & Beta-Amyrin, Beta-sitosterol, Fumaric acid, Mallic acid, Citric acid, Quercetin, Kaempferol, Calcium sulphate, Calcium oxalate.

Folk Use: Wound healing.

Use in literature: Leaves – Diarrhoea, disuria, dysentery, polyuria, tuberculosis, ulcers.

Leaves (Externally applied)- Bleeding, calculii, cuts, ulcers, wounds.

169. *Lannea coromandelica* Merr. (Anacardiaceae)

Syn.: *L. grandis* Engl.

Distribution: Common in dry deciduous forests. Bhopal, Hosahangabad, Indore, Jabalpur, Mandla, Seoni, Shivpuri.

Botany: Trees, leaves pinnately compound; flowers Purplish; ripe fruits red drupes. Flowering & Fruiting: February-May.

Medicinal parts: Bark

Chemical constituents: Bark contains-β-Sitosterol, Physcion, Phlobatannins, Physcion anthranol-B.

Leaves contain – Ellagic acid, Quercetin, β-Sitosterol, Rutin, Leucocyandin, Leucodelphinidin.

Flowers contain – Quercetin, Iso-quercitrin, Morin, Ellagic acid.

Folk Use: Bone fracture

Use in literature:

Bark – Cuts, Diarrhoea, Dysentery, Gout, Wounds, Heart complaints, Opthalmia, Stomatitis, Ulcers.

Leaves – Bodyache, Elephantitis, Inflammation, Swellings.

170. *Lantana camara* L. (Verbenaceae)

Distribution: On roadsides and forest margins. Balaghat, Chhatarpur, Damoh, Dhar, Hosahangabad, Indore, Narsimhapur, Panna, Satna, Shivpuri, Sidhi, Tikamgarh.

Botany: Prickly shrubs, prickles hooked. Leaves ovate or ovate-oblong. Flowers multicoloured, orange-yellow, pink or red. Drupes globose, black when ripe.

Flowering & Fruiting**:** Throughout the Year.

Medicinal Parts: Whole plant.

Chemical constituents: Plant contains Essential oil.

Leaves contain Lantanine, lantadene, arachidic acid, linoleic acid, myristic acid, palmitic acid, citral, eugenol, furfural, geraniol, linalool, Alpha- amyrin, Beta- sitosterol. Lantanin acid, lantadene- A & B. verbascoses & lantanane.

Folk Use: Rheumatism, Ringworm

Use in literature: Fistula, malaria, rheumatim, wounds.

171. *Lawsonia inermis* L. (Lythraceae)

Syn.: *L. alba* Lamk. Egyptian

Vern.: Mehndi.

Distribution: Almost throughout the State; usually planted as hedge.

Botany: Much branched shrubs, with broadly lanceolate leaves and creamish, fragrant flowers. Capsules globose.

Flowering & Fruiting**:** May – November.

Medicinal Parts: Leaves, Stem Bark, flowers, fruits.

Chemical constituents: Leaves contain Heena dye, Hanno – tannic acid, tannin, olive green resin.

Folk Use: Boils Burn, Headache, Piles, Rheumatism, Snake bite

Use in literature: Amenorrhoea, bronchitis, cough, haemorrhage, headache, leprosy, leucoderma, lumbago, scabies, skin diseases, stomatitis, ulcer.

172. *Leptadenia reticulata* Wight & Arn. (Asclepiadaceae)

Distribution: In Sal forests, mostly on red morrum or sandy soil. Hoshangabad.

Botany: Perennial climbers, with green or yellow flowers and follicle fruits. Flowering & Fruiting: July-April.

Medicinal Parts: Leaves.

Folk Use: Typhoid.

Use in literature: Leaves/Roots – Skin affections.

Plant – Habitual abortion.

173. *Leucas cephalotes* (Roth.) Spreng. (Lamiaceae)

Syn.: L. aspera (Willd.) Link.

Vern.: Dhurpi sag.

Distribution: Amidst grasses in forest clearings and in cultivated fields. Balaghat, Betul, Chhatarpur, Damoh, Dhar, Sagar, Satna, Seoni, Sidhi, Tikamgarh, W. Nimar.

Botany: Erect, hispid herbs, with ovate, crenate-serrate leaves. Flowers white, in large, globose terminal heads. Calyx-tube bent, mouth produced on the upper side, villous within. Nutlets obovoid-oblong.

Flowering & Fruiting: August-April.

Medicinal Parts: Whole plant, flowers.

Chemical constituents: Plant contains B- Sitosterol, flavonoides, glycosides, glucose, alkaloids, baballenic acid, aromatic oil.

Folk Use: Cold, Cough

Use in literature: Asthma, bronchitis, cold, cough, dyspepsia, eruptions, eye complaint, headache, inflammation, jaundice, leucoma, paralysis, scabies, skin diseases, snake bite, swelling.

174. *Limonia acidissima* L. (Rutaceae)

Syn.: *Feronia elephantum* Corr.; *F. limonia* (L.) Swing.

Vern.: Kabit.

Distribution: Hoshangabad, Panna.

Botany: Medium sized trees, armed spine. Leaves imparipinnate, with 3-9 leaflets. Flowers pentamerous, yellowish. Fruit globose, with woody rind.

Flowering & Fruiting: February– October.

Medicinal Parts: Fruits.

Chemical constituents: Fruits contain Riboflavine, vitamin – C pectin, Iron, phosphorus.

Leaves contain Volatile oil (Estragol).

Folk Use: Boils, Dysentery

Use in literature: Fruits – Asthma, biliousness, blood diseases, cough, dysentery, earache, heart diseases, hiccough, leucorrhoea, ophthalmia, throat diseases, tumour, vomiting.

Seed – Headache, heart diseases.

Leaf – Dysentery, hiccough, vomiting.

175. *Madhuca indica* Gmel. (Sapotaceae)

Syn.: *M. longifolia* (Koenig) Mach. Var. *latifolia* Chev.; *Bassia latifolia* Roxb.

Vern.: Mahua.

Distribution: Common throughout the state on roadsides, near villages and in dry mixed deciduous forests. Chhatarpur, Damoh, Shivpuri, Sidhi.

Botany: Large, deciduous trees, with elliptic-obovate leaves and white flowers in axillary fascicles. Berries ovoid.

Flowering & Fruiting: April – June.

Medicinal Parts: Flower, Fruit, Leaves, Bark, Seed oil.

Chemical constituents: Flowers Sugar, cellulose.

Seeds Oil.

Folk Use: Bone fracture, Muscular pain, Rheumatism, Snake bite, Sprain, Tonic, Wound

Use in literature: Plant – Biliousness, burning sensation, ulcer.

Bark – Bone fracture, leprosy, ulcer, wounds.

Flower – Biliousness, burning sensation, ear complaint, heart diseases.

Fruits – blood diseases, bronchitis, heart diseases.

Seed oil – Burning sensation.

176. *Mangifera indica* L. (Anacardiaceae)

Vern.: Aam.

Distribution: Commonly planted throughout the State. Bhopal, Chhindwada, Damoh, Hosahangabad, Jabalpur, Mandla, Raisen, Rewa, Shahdol, Shivpuri.

Botany: Evergreen trees, with oblong-lanceolate leaves and polygamous flowers in panicles. Stamens and style solitary. Drupes yellow when ripe.

Flowering & Fruiting: Febuary – June.

Medicinal Parts: Leaves, bark, flower, fruits, seed, gum.

Chemical constituents: Mangiferin, Amino acids, Gallotanin, Gallic acid, Ethylgallati, Isoquercetin, β- Sitosterol, Riboflavin, Vitamin- C, citronellal, Deterpene, Geraniol, Limonene, mangiferol, Mangiferon, Nerol & Tannine, Vitamin- A, Ascorbic acid, protein, fat, carbohydrate, Calcium, phosphorous, Iron, fructose, sucrose, glucose.

Folk Use: Diabetes, Diarrhoea, Dysentery, Sun stroke

Use in literature: Unripe fruits – Biliousness, blood impurities, dysentery, throat trouble, ulcer, urinary dischargers, vaginal trouble.

Flower – Biliousness, blood diseases, bronchitis, dysentery, leucorrhoea, urinary discharges.

Ripe fruit – Blood impurities, heart trouble, ulcers, urinary discharges.

Seed – Dysentery, vomiting.

Seed oil – Stomatitis.

177. *Martynia annua* L. (Martyniaceae)

Vern.: Bicchu.

Distribution: In wastelands. Balaghat, Damoh, Dhar, Hosahangabad, Indore, Mandla, Panna, Ratlam, Rewa, Sagar, Satna, Sidhi.

Botany: Glandular pubescent herbs, with fistular stem, ovate-cordate leaves & drooping, pinkish-white flowers. Fruits woody, beetle-shaped, hooked at the tip. Flowering & Fruiting: August-November.

Medicinal Parts: Fruit, Root, Seed.

Chemical Constituents: Leaves – Chlorogenic acid.

Seeds – Pale Yellow semi drying oil, Fatty oil: Fatty acids of the fatty oil are Palmitic, Stearic, arachidic, Oleic acid, Linoleic etc.

Fruits – Fatty oil: Fatty acids of the fatty oil are Plamitic, Stearic, Oleic acid, Linoleic acid.

Folk Use: Cold, Scorpion sting, Snake bite

Use in literature: Fruits – Inflammation.

Leaves – Epilepsy, Sore throat.

178. *Melia azedarach* L. (Meliaceae)

Vern.: Bakayan.

Distribution: Usually planted throughout Madhya Pradesh.

Botany: Trees, with 1 to 3-pinnate leaves and liliac flowers. Drupes 5-located, each locule 1-seeded.

Flowering & Fruiting: April– May.

Medicinal Parts: Flowers.

Chemical constituents: Plant contains Azaridine, Bakayanin, Bakalactone, Morgosine, Azadirone, Azadiradione, Orchinol, Ochinine, Ochinolal, Nimbolinin, Nimbolidins, Triterpene, Meliacins, Sendanins, Melianol, Melianone, Lupeol, β- stiosterol, Cataechin, Vanillin, Cinnamic acid, Cystine, Serin, Arginine, Glycine, Glutomic acid, Leucine, Threonine, Methionine.

Folk Use: Kill lice

Use in literature: Root – Amenorrhoea, asthma, burning sensation, cough, diabetes, dysenetery, fever, general debility helmintic, leprosy, leucoderma, lumbago, sciatica, skin diseases, ulcer, vomit, wound.

Leaf – Amenorrhoea, bronchitis, cardiac diseases, cough, hysteria, inflammation, leprosy, scabies.

Seed – Fever, helmintic, typhoid.

Flower – Dysenetery, fever.

179. *Mentha spicata* L. (Lamiaceae)

Syn.: *Mentha vidrdis* L.

Vern.: Podina.

Distribution: Cultivated throughout the state as field crops.

Botany: Aromatic, creeping or ascending herbs. Leaves ovate or ovate-elliptic. Flowers purplish. Flowering & Fruiting: June-July.

Medicinal Parts: Leaves.

Chemical Constituents: Diosmetin, Diosmin from leaves. Essential oil contains Carvacrol, L-carvone, Dihydrocarveol, Limonene, Dipentene and Esters.

Folk Use: Dyspepsia, Vomiting

Use in literature: Leaves – Bronchtis, Fever.

180. *Merremia emarginata* (Burm. f.) Hall. f. (Convolvulaceae)

Syn.: *M. gangetica* (L.) Cuf.; *Ipomoea reniformis* Choisy.

Distribution In wastelands, along edges of fields and on sandy slopes. Bhopal, Chhatarpur, Damoh, Seoni.

Botany: A creeping perennial herb rooting at the nodes; Leaves simple, long stalked, reniform or ovate-cordate, flowers yellow, axillary on 1-3 flowered, very short peduncles; fruits subglbose capsules with 2-4 glabrous light brown seeds.

Flowering & Fruiting**:** December-March.

Medicinal Parts: Whole plant.

Chemical constituents: Seeds contain Caffic acid, ferrulic acid, sinapic acid, p-coumaric acid.

Folk Use: Fever, Snake bite

Use in literature: Plant – Anaemia, cardiac diseases, fever, leucoderma, strangury.

181. *Merremia tridentata* (L.) Hallier f ssp. *tridentata* (Convolvulaceae)

Syn.: *Ipomoea tridentata* (L.) Roth.

Distribution: In wastelands & river beds.

Botany: A small glabrous perennial herb with many decumbent stems from a small woody rootstock. Leaves sessile. Flowers axillary, peduncles wiry, 1-3-flowered; pedicels, sub-clavate. Sepals elliptic, glabrous. Capsules ovoid, glabrous, 2-celled. Seeds dark, glabrous. Flowering & Fruiting: September-December.

Medicinal Parts: Root.

Folk Use: Rheumatism

Use in literature: Plant – General debility, Haemorrhoids, Inflammation, Inflammation,Uropathy.

182. *Mimusops hexandra* (Roxb.) Dub. (Sapotaceae)

Syn.: *Manilkara hexandra* (Roxb.) Dub.

Vern.: Khirni.

Distribution: Along roadsides and near strems. Chhatarpur, Damoh, Dhar, Hosahangabad, Indore, Panna, Raisen, Rewa, Sagar, Satna.

Botany: Small trees; bark rough, grey; Leaves oblong, elliptic or elliptic-ovate; flowers white, in fascicles of 2-6 and from the axils of follen leaves; fruits oblond-ellipsoid, reddish-yellow when ripe; seeds ovoid, reddish-brown, shining.

Flowering & Fruiting: September-December.

Medicinal Parts: Root

Folk Use: Headache

Use in literature: Fruit – Biliousness, hallucinations, heart diseases, leprosy, loss of consciousness.

183. *Mitragyna parvifolia* (Roxb.) Korth. (Rubiaceae)

Syn.: *Stephegyne parvifolia* Korth.

Vern.: Karam, Mundi.

Distribution: Balaghat, Bhopal, Chhatarpur, Damoh, Hosahangabad, Indore, Jabalpur, Mandla, Morena, Narsimhapur, Panna, Rewa, Sagar, Satna, Seoni, Shahdol, Shivpuri, Sidhi, Tikamgarh.

Botany: Trees, with panduriform or ovate to suborbicular leaves. Flowers in heads, greenish-yellow, with mitriform stigma. Capsules oblong-ellipsoid, 10-ribbed.

Flowering & Fruiting: August– January.

Medicinal Parts: Root, bark, leaves.

Folk Use: Colic, Cuts, Fever, Jaundice

Use in literature: Root & bark – Colic, fever.

Leaf – Colic, dyspepsia, erysipelas, fever, flatulence, inflammation, leprosy, skin diseases, wound.

184. *Momordica charantia* L. (Cucurbitaceae)

Vern.: Karela.

Distribution: Commonly cultivated throughout the State.

Botany: Monoecious climbers, with 5 to 7-lobed leaves and yellow flowers. Bracts of male flowers born about or below the middle of peduncle. Fruits muricate-tuberculate.

Flowering & Fruiting: July- October.

Medicinal Parts: Fruit.

Chemical constituents: Plant contains Aromatic essential oil, Carotene, Glucoside, saponine, Momoridicine alkaloid, charantin (non nitrogenous substance).

Folk Use: Rheumatism

Use in literature: Leaf – Burning sensation, constipation, fever, helminthiasis.

Fruits – Asthma, burning sensation, colic, constipation, cough, diabetes, fever gout, helminthiases, inflammation, leprosy, skin diseases, ulcer, wound.

Seed – Obstructions of the liver & spleen, ulcer.

185. *Momordica dioica Roxb.* ex Willd. (Cucurbitaceae)

Vern.: Jangli Karela.

Distribution: Commonly throughout the State.

Botany: Perinnial, dioecious climbers, with tuberous roots. Leaves ovate, entire or 3 to 5-lobed. Flowers yellow. Fruits ovoid, beaked, densely echinate with soft spines.

Flowering & Fruiting: June – October.

Medicinal Parts: Fruits.

Chemical constituents: Plant contains Alkaloids, mangenese.

Folk Use: Diabetes, Fever

Use in literature: Root – Headache, jaundice, urinary calculi.

Leaf – Asthma, bronchitis, fever, hiccough, piles.

Fruits – Asthma, biliousness, bronchitis, fever, heart trouble, leprosy, tumour, urinary discharges.

186. *Morinda pubescens* J.E. Smith. (Rubiaceae)

Syn.: *M. coreia* Buch-Ham.; *M. tinctoria* Roxb.

Distribution: Balaghat, Indore, Morena, Satna, Seoni.

Botany: Moderate sized deciduous trees, with White flowers & drupe fruits. Flowering & Fruiting: March-August.

Medicinal Parts: Seed oil.

Chemical Constituents: Root – Morindone and its Glucoside Morindine; Damnacanthal, Nordamnacanthal, β-Sitosterol, Anthragallol-2-3-dimethyl ether, Soranjidol, Ibericin, Morindone-6-Primeveroside.

Leaves – Campesterol, Stigmasterol, β-sitosterol, Ursolic acid.

Folk Use: Rheumatism

Use in literature: Root – Boils, Dysentery, General debility, Haemorrhages, Inflammation.

Leaves – Diarrhoea, Dyspepsia, Gaotropathy, Gout, Inflammation, Ulcerative stomatitis, Wounds.

187. *Moringa oleifera* Lam. (Moringaceae)

Syn.: *M. pterygosperma* Gaertn.

Vern.: Munga, Sahjan.

Distribution: Planted in the vicinity of Villages. Guna, Gwalior, Hosahangabad, Indore, Jabalpur, Mandla, Raisen, Seoni, Shivpuri, Sidhi.

Botany: Small trees, with 3-pinnate leaves and creamy-yellow or white flowers without red streaks on petals. Fruits slender, 3-gonous, 9-ribbed.

Flowering & Fruiting: February-June.

Medicinal Parts: Root, bark, leaf, seed.

Chemical constituents: Root bark contains Alkaloids, Moringine, Moringinine, Spirochin, Ptrigospermine.

Leaf & fruits contain Vitamin- A, Nicotinic acid, Ascorbic acid, Vitamin- B, fatty acid.

Flower & fruits contain Amino acids, glucose & sucrose, Citric acid, Malic acid, Succinic acid, Fumaric acid, Oxalic acid.

Folk Use: Asthma, Pain, Swelling, Typhoid,

Use in literature: Root – Amenorrhoea, asthma, bronchitis, cough, diarrohoea, dysentery, dyspepsia, epilepsies, fever, hysteria, inflammation, otalgia, paralysis.

Bark – Ringworm

Leaf – Helminthiasis, inflammation, scurvy, tumours, wounds.

Seed – Fever, inflammation, neuralgia.

188. *Mucuna pruriens* (L.) DC. (Papilionaceae)

Syn.: *M. prurita* Hook.

Vern.: Kemuch.

Distribution: Climbing on Shrubs and trees on road sides and forest edges. Balaghat, Bhopal, Damoh, Dhar, Gwalior, Hosahangabad,

Indore, Jabalpur, Mandla, Panna, Raisen, Seoni, Shahdol, Sidhi, W. Nimar.

Botany: Twining herbs, with 3-foliolate leaves and purple flowers in racemes. Pods densely bristly slightly curved at both ends.

Flowering & Fruiting: September-May.

Medicinal Parts: Root, leaf, seed.

Chemical constituents: Seed contains Carbohydrates, Steroids, Phenols, Glycosides, Tannin, Aluminium, Iron, Zinc, Calcium, Magnessium, Potessium.

Folk Use: Aphrodisiac, Fever

Use in literature: Root – Amenorrhoea, constipation, dropsy, dysmenorrhoea, elephantiasis, fever, helminthiasis, ulcers.

Leaf – General debility, helminthiasis, inflammation, ulcers.

Sour – General deblility, gonorrhoea, sterility.

189. *Murraya paniculata* (L.) Jack. (Rutaceae)

Syn.: *M. exotica* L.

Vern.: Kamini.

Distribution: Bhopal, Damoh.

Botany: A small evergreen shrub or tree; leaves pinnately compound; flowers white, fragrant; fruits red berries.

Flowering & Fruiting: October-April.

Medicinal Parts: Leaves.

Chemical constituents: Leaves contain – Phebalocin, Heptamethoxy flavon.

Fruits contain – Paniculatin, coumarin.

Flower contains – Scopoletin, glucose.

Roots contain – Alkaloids: Noracronycine & skimmiacine.

Folk Use: Diarrhoea, Dysentery, Joint pain

Use in literature: Leaves – Diarrhoea, dropsy, dysentery.

Root bark – Cough, hysteria, rheumatism.

190. *Nelumbo nucifera* Gaertn. (Nymphaeaceae)

Syn.: *Nelumbium speciosum* Willd.; *Nelumbium nelumbo* Druce.

Vern.: Kamal.

Distribution: In old tanks and Marshes. Damoh, Indore, Mandla, Sagar.

Botany: Perennial, rhizomatous aquatic herbs; leaves orbicular, peltate, 32-60 cm across; flowers white to pink, solitary on long axillary peduncles, sepals caducous; petals many seriate; carpels many, free, embeded in an obconical receptacle.

Flowering & Fruiting: April-January.

Medicinal Parts: Rhizome, Seed.

Chemical constituents: Rhizome contain Glucose, tannin, fat, resin, metarbin & an alkaloid – Nelumbine.

Folk Use: Dyspepsia, Skin diseases

Use in literature: Stem – Helminthiasis, leprosy, skin diseases, vomit.

Root – Cough, diarrhoea, dyspepsia, leucoderma, small pox, spermatorrhoea.

Leaf – Burning sensation, fever, leprosy.

Flowers – Bronchitis, cholera, cough, diarrohea, fever.

Fruit & Seeds – Burning sensation, fever, leprosy, leucorrhoea, pruritus, vomit.

191. *Nerium indicum* Mill. (Apocynaceae)

Syn.: *N. odorum* Soland.; *N. oleander* L.

Vern.: Kaner.

Distribution: Ornamental, cultivated in gardens. Chhatarpur, Damoh, Dhar, Rewa, Satna, Shivpuri, Sidhi, W. Nimar.

Botany: Evergreen shrubs, with linear-elliptic leaves and white or red flowers in cymes.

Flowering & Fruiting: Throughout the year.

Medicinal Parts: Leaves.

Chemical constituents: Root bark contains Neriodorin, Nerioderin, Karabin, Glucoside (Odorin).

Leaf contains Oleandrin, Neriodin, Ursolic acid, Adynerin.

Flower contains Parafin, Benzyl alcohol, Compesterol, stigma sterol, fatty acids.

Folk Use: Skin diseases

Use in literature: Root – Asthma, leprosy, pruritus, ulcers.

Leaf – Haemorrhoids, scabies.

192. *Nicotiana tabacum* L. (Solanaceae)

Syn.: *N. macrophylla* Lehm.; *N. auriculata* Bert.

Vern.: Tambaku.

Distribution: Widely cultivated throughout the State and also as wild along the drains and on abandoned hill tops. Damoh, Hosahangabad, Mandla, Sidhi.

Botany: Glandular-pubescent herbs, with Pinkish flowers and ovate capsules.

Flowering & Fruiting: Septamber-April.

Medicinal Parts: Leaves.

Chemical constituents: Leaves Nicotine alkaloid.

Folk Use: Hydocele

Use in literature: Leaves – Asthma, bronchitis, dyspepsia, flatlulence, haemorrhages, helminthiasis, inflammations, scabies, skin diseases, ulcers.

193. *Nyctanthes arbor-tristis* L. (Oleaceae)

Vern.: Harsinghar.

Distribution: Common in dry mixed deciduous forests and hill slopes. Balaghat, Chhatarpur, Damoh, Dhar, Indore, Jabalpur, Mandla, Narsimhapur, Panna, Rewa, Sagar, Satna, Seoni, Sidhi, W. Nimar.

Botany: Large shrubs, with 4-angled branches and ovate or ovate-lanceolate leaves. Flowers white to orange, fragrant. Capsule orbicular, compressed.

Flowering & Fruiting: September-January.

Medicinal Parts: Leaves.

Chemical constituents: Leaf & stem contains Beta- Sitosterol, Nyctanthic acid, Iridoid, Glycosides- Arbortristosides A, B, C, D & E Glucomannan, Glycerides of Lignocetric, Linocetric, Myristic acid, Oleic acid, palmitic acid, Stearic acid (In Seeds), As tragalin, Nictoflorin, Nyctanthoside, Arborsides, Ascorbic acid, Carotene, Glucose, Fructose, Manitol.

Folk Use: Rheumatism, Sciatica

Use in literature: Leaf – Baldness, bronchitis, constipation, cough, dyspepsia, fever, helminthiasis, inflammation, pruritus, sciatica.

Seed – Scurvy.

194. *Nymphaea nauchali* Burm f. (Nymphaeaceae)

Syn.: *N. lotus* Hook. f. & Thoms non L.; *N. pubescens* Willd.; *N. rubra* Roxb. ex Salisb.

Vern.: Neelkamal.

Distribution: In tanks and marshes. Balaghat, Damoh, Gwalior, Indore, Jabalpur, Rewa, Sagar, Satna.

Botany: Rhizomatous perennial floating herbs; leaves large, 15-20 cm across; orbicular, regularly sinuately, toothed, densely tomentose beneath, flowers white to blue about 10 cm across.

Flowering & Fruiting: May-November.

Medicinal Parts: Rhizomes.

Folk Use: Dysentery, Dyspepsia

Use in literature: Rhizome – Diarrhoea, dysentery, dyspepsia, debility, gonorrhoea.

Seed – Diarrhoea, dispepsia.

195. *Ocimum basilicum* L. (Lamiaceae)

Syn.: *O. caryophyllantum* Roxb.; *O. pilosum* Willd.

Vern.: Marwa.

Distribution: In wastelands, forest floor and nearby habitations. Balaghat, Betul, Chhatarpur, Gwalior, Indore, Jabalpur, Rewa, Satna, Seoni, Sidhi, Tikamgarh.

Botany: An erect branching herb. Stem and branches green or purplish. Leaves ovate-lanceolate, entire or toothed. Flowers whitish-pink or purplish, in whorls on simple or branched racemes. Corolla glabrous or variously pubiscent. Nutlets black, pitted.

Flowering & Fruiting: July-April.

Medicinal Parts: Leaves.

Chemical constituents: Plant contains Ocimene, Methyl chavicol, Ceneol, Linoalool, Pinene- Camphor terpin hydrate, aromatic oil.

Folk Use: Ringworm

Use in literature: Affections, agalactia, amenorrhoea, asthma, bronchitis, cardiac debility, colic, cough, diarrohoea, dysentery, dyspepsia, fever flatulence, helminthiasis, inflammation, leucoderma, neuralgia, otalgia, pruritus, rheumatism, ringworm, skin diseases, spasmodic, vomit.

196. *Ocimum canum* Sims. (Lamiaceae)

Syn.: *O. americanum* Aut. non L.

Vern.: Jungli tulsi.

Distribution: In wastelands, forest floor, and nearby habitations. Chhatarpur, Indore, Mandla, Narsimhapur, Rewa, Satna, Seoni.

Botany: Herbs or undershrubs, with ovate-lanceolate or ovate-oblong leaves. Flowers white, whorled in long racemes. Calyx-tube hirsute-annulate within. Nutlets ovoid.

Flowering & Fruiting**:** August-March.

Medicinal Parts: Leaves.

Chemical constituents: Plant contains Glycosides, alkaloids, tannins, savonin, volatile oil, vitamin- C, carotene.

Seed contains Green coloured oil, systosterol, fatty acid, palmitic acid, oleic acid, linoleic acid, linolenic acid, mucilage.

Folk Use: Fever

Use in literature: Antispasmodic, asthma, diabetes, itching, malaria, ringworm, spermatorrhoes, tuberculosis, urino- genital diseases.

197. *Ocimum gratissimum* L. (Lamiaceae)

Vern.: Ramtulasi.

Distribution: In Wastelands and along roadsides. Balaghat, Damoh, Dhar, Indore, Jabalpur, Seoni.

Botany: Tall, strongly aromatic shrubs; leaves ovate-lanceolate, tapering at base and decurrent on the petiole; flowers white, in verticillasters; nutlets 2 mm across.

Flowering & Fruiting**:** September– March.

Medicinal Parts: Leaves.

Chemical constituents: Leaves contain Essential oil, steroids, ascorbic acid, glycosides, saponins, tannins.

Folk Use: Rheumatism

Use in literature: Colic, cough, disuria, erysipelas, fever, gonorrhoea, inflammation, leucoderma, polyuria, seminal debility, skin diseases, strangury, vomiting.

198. *Ocimum sanctum* L. (Lamiaceae)

Syn.: *O. tenuiflorum* Sensu keng.

Vern.: Tulsi.

Distribution: Inwaste lands and under cultivation throughout the State. Chhatarpur, Damoh, Indore, Panna, Rewa, Sidhi, Tikamgarh.

Botany: A much branched, woody herb. Stems and branches clothed with soft spreading purplish hairs. Leaves opposite-decussate, ovate, elliptic-oblong, entire or crenate serrate, hairy, minutely gland dotted. Flowers purplish-pink, whorld, in racemes, often forming panicles. Nutlets broad ellipsoid, smooth.

Flowering & Fruiting: Most part of the year.

Medicinal Parts: Leaves.

Chemical constituents: Plant contains Essential oil Eugenol, Eugenol methyl ether, carvacrol, Caryophyllene, Ursolic acid, Apigenin, Luteolin, Ascorbic acid, Carotene, Alkaloid, Glycosides, Saponins & Tannins.

Folk Use: Asthma, Cold, Cough, Earache, Ringworm

Use in literature: Asthma, bronchitis, hiccough, leucoderma, lumbago, otalgia, ringworm, skin diseases, urino- genital disorders, vomit.

199. *Oldenlandia corymbosa* L. (Rubiaceae)

Vern.: Dhaman-paper.

Syn.: *Hedyotis corymbosa* (L.) Lam.

Distribution: Balaghat, Bhopal, Chhatarpur, Damoh, Gwalior, Hosahangabad, Jabalpur, Mandla, Narsimhapur, Panna, Ratlam, Sagar, Seoni, Shivpuri, Sidhi.

Botany: A small herbs; leaves subsessile, linear-lanceolate, acute, recurved and hairy margins, stipules membranous with few bristles; flowers white, small on solitary long peduncle; fruits globose capsule.

Flowering & Fruiting: September-April.

Medicinal Parts: Whole plant.

Chemical constituents: Whole plant – Alkaloids-Biflorine & Biflorone; Sodium, Potassium, Calcium, Chloride; caffeine, fumaric acid, oleanolic acid, ursolic acid, methyl ether.

Folk Use: Burning sensation, Fever, Jaundice

Use in literature: Bronchitis, fever, jaundice, liver disorders, malaria fever, measles.

200. *Opuntia elatior* Mill. (Cactaceae)

Syn.: *O. nigricans* Haw.

Vern.: Naagphani.

Distribution: In waste places, along roadsides & a hedges around cultivated fields.

Botany: Spreading bush, with flat, succulent, jointed, obovate branches having several straight spines on each cushion. Flowering & Fruiting: March-Septeember.

Medicinal Parts: Pulp.

Chemical Constituents: Flower contains Glycoside of Isorhamnetin and Quercertain and Glucoside narcissi. Isolation of Isoquercitrin, β-sitosterol, Opintiol. A Polysaccharide contains Galactose and Arabinose from Pods.

Folk Use: Inflammation

Use in literature: Fruits – Gonorrhoea, Whooping Cough.

201. *Oroxylum indicum* (L.) Vent. (Bignoniaceae)

Syn.: *Bignonia indica* L.; *Calosanthes indica* Blume.

Vern.: Arlu.

Distribution: In mixed forests. Chhatarpur, Seoni.

Botany: Trees, with 2 to 3-pinnate leaves. Flowers in racemes; corolla fleshy; stamens 5. Capsules elongate, compressed.

Flowering & Fruiting: June – March.

Medicinal Parts: Leaves.

Chemical constituents: Root bark contain Oroxylin- A bitter glycoside, acrid substance, pectin chrysie, baicalein oil.

Seed contain Tetuin, flavin, glucoside, fatty acid & Amino acids.

Bark contain Sodium salicilate.

Folk Use: Fever, Rheumatism

Use in literature: Root – Asthma, bronchitis, colic, cough, diarrhoea, dropsy, dysentery, dyspepsia, fever, flatulence, gout, hiccough, helmintic, inflammation, leucoderma, neuralgia, vomit.

Leaf – Flatulence, ulcers.

Fruits – Bronchitis, cardiac disorder, haemorrhoids, helminthiasis.

202. *Ougeinia oojeinesis* (Roxb.) Hochr. (Papilionaceae)

Syn.: *O. dalbergioides* Benth.

Vern.: Tinsa.

Distribution: In mixed forests. Balaghat, Bhopal, Chhindwara, Gwalior, Indore, Jabalpur, Mandla, Panna, Raisen, Sagar, Seoni, Shahdol.

Botany: A medium sized deciduous trees, with liliac or White flowers and flat pods. Flowering & Fruiting: February-June.

Medicinal Parts: Bark.

Chemical Constituents: Bark contains – Triterpenoids as lupeol, Betulin, β-amyrin & Hydroxylupeol.

Folk Use: Body swellings, Boils

Use in literature: Bark – Anaemia, Burning sensation, Diarrhoea, Dysentery, Fever, Inflammation, Leprosy, Leucoderma, General debility, Gonorrhoea, Ulcers.

203. *Oxalis corniculata* L. (Oxalidaceae)

Vern.: Amrulsak.

Distribution: Balaghat, Hosahangabad, Jabalpur, Mandla, Narsimhapur, Panna, Sagar, Seoni, Sidhi.

Botany: Procumbent, apprised hairy herbs; leaves digitately 3-foliolate; leaflets subsessile cuneate or acute at base, appressed hairy; flowers yellow, 2-8 in umbellate clusters; capsule oblong, narrowed to the apex, pubescent; seeds transversely ribbed.

Flowering & Fruiting: January-December.

Medicinal Parts: Leaves, Whole plant.

Chemical constituents: Plant contains Malic acid, Tarteric acid, Citric acid, Potassium Oxalate.

Folk Use: Diarrhoea, Fertility, Menstrual disorders

Use in literature: Amenorrhoea, anemia, diarrhoea, dysentery, dysmenorrhoea, dyspepsia, fever, haemorrhages, scurvy, warts.

204. *Pandanus fascicularis* Lamk. (Pandanaceae)

Syn.: *P. tectorius* Auct. Non Park.; *P. odoratissimus* L. f.

Vern.: Kevda.

Distribution: Common along streams and paddy fields.

Botany: Much-branched, small trees, with aerial roots. Leaves drooping spirally arranged, ensiform, with recurved marginal spines. Flowers white, sweet scented. Fruits woody, yellowish-brown.

Flowering & Fruiting: February-September.

Medicinal Parts: Root, leaf, flower.

Chemical constituents: Plant contains Physcion, Circilineol, Circilineol, n- tricontanol, β- stiosterol, stigmasterol, compesterol, Daucosterol, Palmitic acid, Stearic acid.

Folk Use: Miscarriages, Rheumatism, Scabies

Use in literature: Root – Abortion, colic, diabetes, dyspepsia, fever, flatulence, general debility, leprosy, otalgia, sterility, ulcers, wounds.

Leaf – Leprosy, leucoderma, scabies, small pox, syphilis, tumours.

Flower – Leucoderma, otalgia, pruritus.

205. *Pergularia daemia* (Forsk.) Chiov. (Asclepiadaceae)

Syn.: *P. extensa* (Jacq.) R. Br.; *Daemia extensa* (Jacq.) R. Br.

Vern.: Sadowani.

Distribution: Climber on roadside shrubs and trees. Balaghat, Bhopal, Chhatarpur, Damoh, E. Nimar, Indore, Mandla, Rewa, Sagar, Satna, Shahdol, ShivpuriTikamgarh

Botany: Twining undershrubs, with cordate-ovate and acuminate leaves. Flowers yellowish-green, in drooping, corymbose cymes; corolla salver- shaped. Follicles echinate.

Flowering & Fruiting: May-July.

Medicinal Parts: Whole plant.

Folk Use: Diarrhoea, Asthma, Rheumatism

Use in literature: Amenorrhoea, asthma, cough, dysmenorrhoea, fever, inflammation, leucoderma..

206. *Phaseolus mungo* (L.) Mant. (Papilionaceae)

Syn.: *Vigna mungo* (L.) Hepper.

Vern.: Urd.

Distribution: Commonly cultivated. Chhindwara, Hoshangabad, Rewa, Sagar, Shivpuri.

Botany: Trailing, hispid herbs, with 3-foliolate leaves & yellow flowers. Pods linear, turgid. Flowering & Fruiting: August-November.

Medicinal Parts: Seed.

Chemical Constituents: The plant contains Albuminoids, Starch and Oil.

Seed contains Saponin I, II & III. It contains Genistein, □-Hydroxygenistein, Dalbergioidin etc.

Folk Use: Fever

Use in literature: Seeds – Asthma, Cough, Dysentery, Diarrhoea, Dyspepsia, Paralysis, Piles, Rheumatism.

207. *Phyllanthus emblica* L. (Euphorbiaceae)

Syn.: *Emblica officinalis* Gaertn.

Vern.: Amla.

Distribution: Common in mixed forests throughout the state, also planted for its edible fruits.

Botany: Large, deciduous trees, with distichous, linear-oblong leaves. Flowers greenish-yellow, in fascicles on leafless branches. Fruits globose, fleshy; seeds bony.

Flowering & Fruiting: March-December.

Medicinal Parts: Root, bark, leaf, fruit.

Chemical constituents: Fruits contain Protein, fats, fibres, Carbohydrates, Vitamin- C, Nicotinic acid, Tannins.

After drying fruits contain Gallic acid, Ellagic acid, Flavin & glucose.

Seed contains Linoleic acid, Linolenic acid, oleic acid.

Folk Use: Stomachache, Skin diseases.

Use in literature: Root bark – Diarrohoea, gonorrhoea, jaundice.

Leaf – Conjunctivitis, diarrohoea, dysentery, dyspepsia, inflammation.

Fruits – Anaemia, asthama, bronchitis, colic, cough, diabetes, diarrohoea, dysentery, dyspepsia, fever, flatulence, haemorrhages, inflammation, jaundice, leprosy, leucorrhoea, menorrhagia, peptie ulcer, skin diseases.

208. *Phyllanthus niruri Auct. non.* L. (Euphorbiaceae)

Syn.: *P. fraternus* Webster.; *P. amarus* Schum. & Thonn.

Vern.: Bhuiamla.

Distribution: Common as weed in gardens, fields and open sandy places near villages. Balaghat, Chhatarpur, Dhar, E. Nimar, Mandla, Panna, Shivpuri, Sidhi, Tikamgarh.

Botany: Erect, annual herbs; stem subterete or obscurely angled; leaves oblong; stipules lanceolate; male flowers 1-3 together; disc lobes 6, glandular; female flowers solitary; perianth segments oblong-spathulate; seeds brown.

Flowering & Fruiting: July- November.

Medicinal Parts: Root, fresh leaves, whole plant.

Chemical constituents: Leaves contain Bitter, Phyllanthin & Hypophyllanthin, Alkaloid, lignas, Vitamin- C, Quercetin, Astrogaln, Querscitrin, Rutin.

Root contains Glucoflavon.

Seed contains Oil which contains- Linoleic & Linolenic acid.

Folk Use: Jaundice

Use in literature: Anaemia, anuria, asthama, biliousness, bronchitis, hiccough, leprosy, menorrhagia, urinary discharges.

209. *Physalis minima* L. (Solanaceae)

Vern.: Ban phutka.

Distribution: In waste lands. Balaghat, Betul, Chhatarpur, Damoh, E. Nimar, Hosahangabad, Mandla, Tikamgarh.

Botany: Erect herbs, with sinuate-dentate leaves. Flowers yellow, axillary, solitary; calyx 5-angled, enclosing yellow berries.

Flowering & Fruiting: August- January.

Medicinal Parts: Leaves, Fruit.

Chemical constituents: Plant contains Steroidal physalin A, B & C. Epaxyphysalin- B, Plamitic acid, stearic acid, Oleic acid, Linoleic acid, Hexadeconoid acid, Epoxy & Hydroxy fatty acid.

Folk Use: Bronchitis, Constipation, Fever

Use in literature: Bronchitis, colic, cough, pruritus, ulcers.

210. *Plumbago zeylanica* L. (Plumbaginaceae)

Vern.: Chitrak.

Distribution: Along roadsides and in forest undergrowth; often planted in gardens. Balaghat, Damoh, Guna, Gwalior, Hosahangabad, Indore, Mandla, Rewa, Sagar, Seoni, Shahdol, Tikamgarh.

Botany: Erect or straggling undershrubs, with ovate-lanceolate leaves and white flowers in panicled racemes. Seed oblong, smooth.

Flowering & Fruiting: August-September.

Medicinal Parts: Root.

Chemical constituents: Plant contains Volatile oil, Chitranone, Alpha & Beta- Amyrin, Lupeol, Taraxasterol, Fructose, Glucose, Ivertase, Protease, Chloroplumbagin, Droserone, Elliptinone, Zeylanone, Zeylinone, Meritone, Catechol, Tannin, Amino acids, Plumbagic acid.

Root contains Plumgagin alkaloids.

Folk Use: Cold, Cough, Headache, Rheumatism

Use in literature: Root – Anaemia, bronchitis, dysentery, inflammation, itching, leucoderma, liver diseases, piles.

211. *Pongamia pinnata* (L.) Pierre (Papilionaceae)

Vern.: Karanj.

Distribution: Generally planted as an avenue tree. Balaghat, Betul, Bhopal, Damoh, Dhar, Hosahangabad, Indore, Jabalpur, Mandla, Panna, Rewa.

Botany: Trees, with imparipinnate leaves. Flowers pinkish-white. Pods obliquely oblong, woody, indehiscent, glabrous.

Flowering & Fruiting: March-February.

Medicinal Parts: Root, bark, leaf, flower, seed.

Chemical constituents: Seed contains Bitter fatty acid oil, Pongamol (Hongay oil) and protein.

Plant contains Alkaloids, tannins, sugar, resin, fatty oil (Karanjin).

Folk Use: Menstrual disorders, Rheumatism, Skin diseases

Use in literature: Root – Gonorrhoea.

Bark – Beriberi, haemorrhoids, ulcers.

Leaf – Cough, diarrohoea, dyspepsia, flatulence, gonorrhoea, leprosy.

Seed – Anaemia, fevers, hydrocele, inflammation, lumbago, otalgia.

Seed oil – Leprosy, lumbago, ulcers, scabies.

212. *Portulaca oleracea* L. (Portulacaceae)

Vern.: Kulfa.

Distribution: In open wastelands. Balaghat, Chhindwara, Gwalior, Indore, Jabalpur, Mandla, Panna, Rewa, Seoni, Shivpuri, Sidhi, Tikamgarh.

Botany: Diffuse herbs, with succulent, obovate-spathulate leaves and yellow flowers. Capsules obovoid.

Flowering & Fruiting: Throughout the year.

Medicinal Parts: Leaves.

Chemical constituents: Plant contains Crude fibres, carbohydrates, calcium, magnesium, phosphorus, Iron, potassium, copper, sulphur, & chlorine.

Folk Use: Injury

Use in literature: Stem & leaves – Diabetes, dysenetery, dyspepsia, gonorrhoea, inflammation, jaundice, otalgia, scurvy, skin diseases, tumours, vomit.

Seed – Burns, dysentery.

213. *Psidium guajava* L. (Myrtaceae)

Vern.: Amrud.

Distribution: Cultivated for its edible fruits, almost in all district.

Botany: A erect, woody shrub or small tree with reddish-brown wood and scaly, brownish bark.Leaves oblong or oblong-elliptic. Flowers on axillary peduncles of 1-3-flowered. Fruits berries.

Flowering & Fruiting: Almost throughout the year, mainly in rainy and cold season.

Medicinal Parts: Fruits.

Chemical constituents: All parts contain Leucocyanidin, Querecetin, β- sitosterol.

Flower & leaves contain Ellagic acid, β- Caryophyllene, Guaijaverin, Umonene, Pinene, Niacin, Vitamin- C & B, Cadinene, β- Cophaene, Curcumene, Farnesene, Citric, Cinnamic, Malic, Oxalic, Quinic, Succinic, Tartaric acids, Riboflavin, Thiamine, Carotene, Tannins, sucrose, Glucose, Fructose, Rhamnose, Starch & Amino acids.

Folk Use: Cold, Constipation, Cough

Use in literature: Root – Diarrhoea, dysentery, haemorrhages, ulcers, vomit.

Leaves – Cholera, diarrhoea, epilepsy, ulcers, vomit, wounds.

Flower – Bronchitis, colic.

Fruits – Colic, diarrhoea, dyspepsia, dysentery, general debility.

214. *Psoralea corylifolia* L. (Papilionaceae)

Vern.: Babchi.

Distribution: Bhopal, E. Nimar, Hosahangabad, Indore, Jabalpur, Raisen, Rewa, Sagar, Seoni, Shivpuri.

Botany: Annual herbs, with simple, suborbicular, gland-dotted leaves. Flowers bluish-purple, packed in upper part of axillary racemes. Pods oblong, 1-seeded.

Flowering & Fruiting: August – November.

Medicinal Parts: Seeds.

Chemical constituents: Seed contains Oil which contain Bakuchi Phenol (This contains Psoralane & Psoradin active Compound), Resin, Volatile oil.

Folk Use: Leprosy, Leucoderma

Use in literature: Leprosy, leucoderma, ulcers.

215. *Pterocarpus marsupium* Roxb. (Papilionaceae)

Vern.: Bijasal.

Distribution: In Sal and Mixed forests, also planted as avenue tree. Balaghat, Bhopal, Chhindwada, Damoh, Gwalior, Hosahangabad, Indore, Jabalpur, Mandla, Raisen, Rewa, Sagar, Seoni, Shahdol, Shivpuri, Sidhi.

Botany: Deciduous trees, with crooked stem and spreading branches. Leaves elliptic or ovate. Flowers pale-yellow, in fusco-paniculate racemes. Pods suborbicular, winged, glabrous.

Flowering & Fruiting: July-March.

Medicinal Parts: Heartwood, leaf, flower, gum.

Chemical constituents: Plant contains Protein, pentosan, mucilage, pterosupin, pseudobaptigenin, liquiritigenin, garbanzol, β- cudesmol, pterostilbene, marsupol, carpusin, propterol, marrsupinol, parsupin, oleanolic acid, tannins & kinotanic acid.

Folk Use: Asthma, Diarrhoea, Dysentery, Fever, Toothache

Use in literature: Heartwood – Asthma, bronchitis, diabetes, diarrhoea, dysentery, cough, elephantiasis, fractures, gout, haemorrhages, inflammation, leprosy, leucoderma, skin diseases.

Leaf – Boils, skin diseases, sores.

Flowers – Fevers.

Gum – Boils, diarrhoea, fever, helmintic, psoriasis, ulcers, wounds.

216. *Pueraria tuberosa* DC. (Papilionaceae)

Vern.: Patal kumhra.

Distribution: On shrubs and small trees in mixed forests. Balaghat, Chhindwada, Hosahangabad, Indore, Jabalpur, Mandla, Shahdol.

Botany: A large spreading tuberous herbaceous twiner with very large tuberous roots; flowers blue or purplish blue in leafless racemes; fruits membranous, flat jointed pods clothed with silky brown hairs.

Flowering & Fruiting: February-April.

Medicinal Parts: Tuberous roots.

Chemical constituents: Hydroxytuberosone, anhydroxytuberosin, 3-O-methylandydrotuberosin, puerarostan, puerarone, daidzein, stigmasterol, puetuberosanol.

Folk Use: Fever, Swelling of joints

Use in literature: Root – Arthritis, burning sensation, constipation, cough, dyspepsia, fevers, leprosy, spermatorrhoea, strangury, tuberculosis.

217. *Punica granatum* L. (Punicaceae)

Vern.: Anar.

Distribution: Planted for its juicy seeds. Chhatarpur, Damoh, Sidhi.

Botany: A large deciduous shrub or small tree, with spiny or thorny branches and dark Grey bark.

Flowering & Fruiting: March-January.

Medicinal Parts: Leaves, Fruits.

Chemical constituents: Bark – Alkaloid-Pelletierine.

Root – Alkaloids, pseudo-pelletierine, pelletierine, isopelletierine, methylpelletierine.

Flowers – Sitosterol, tannins-punicalagin & punicalin.

Fruits – Mannose, galactose, rhamnose, arabinose, glucose, galactouronic acid.

Folk Use: Baldness, Dysentery

Use in literature: Root & Stem bark – Good for tapeworm and for strengthening the gums.

Flowers – Hydrocelc, ulcers, vomiting.

Fruits – Anaemia, bronchitis, otalgia.

Seed – Vomiting, scabies.

218. *Quisqualis indica* L. (Combretaceae)

Syn.: *Q. densiflora* Wall. ex. Mlq.

Vern.: Rangunachi veli

Distribution: Commonly planted in gardens and houses for its attractive flowers. Bhopal, Jabalpur, Mandla, Shivpuri.

Botany: A large, scandent, shrubby and woody vine, with compact terminal spike inflorescence and capsule fruits.

Flowering & Fruiting: Throughout the year.

Medicinal Parts: Leaves, Seeds.

Chemical constituents: Leaves – Trigonelline, L-proline, L-asparagine, quisqualic acid.

Seed oil – Linolenic, oleic, palmitic, stearic, arachidic acids, sterol, fatty acids.

Folk Use: Diarrhoea, Fever, Tonsilitis

Use in literature: Seeds – Diarrhoea, fever, helminthiasis, rickets, ringworm.

Leaves – Colic, constipation, helminthiasis.

219. *Raphanus sativus* L. (Brassicaceae)

Syn.: *R. caudatus* L.

Vern.: Muli.

Distribution: Commonly cultivated as vegetable.

Botany: Annual herbs, with fusiform roots and white or lilac flowers.

Flowering & Fruiting: December-April.

Medicinal Parts: Roots, Leaves, Seeds.

Chemical constituents: Seeds- Glycoside, enzyme, methyl mercaptan, sulforaphene, essential oil.

Folk Use: Menstrual disorders

Use in literature: Root – Colic, diarrhoea, dyspepsia, flatulence, inflammations, leprosy, nausea, skin diseases.

Seeds – Amenorrhoea, cough, dyspepsia, flatulence, paralysis, strangury.

220. *Ricinus communis* L. (Euphorbiaceae)

Vern.: Arandi.

Distribution: Usually cultivated for oil seeds, sometimes found as an escape in wastelands. Chhatarpur, Damoh, Dhar, Seoni, Sidhi, W. Nimar.

Botany: Large shrubs or small trees, with fistular stem and large, palmetly 5 to 10-lobed leaves. Flowers in pyramidal panicles. Capsules globose, spiny, of 3- cocci; seeds caruncled.

Flowering & Fruiting: September-May.

Medicinal Parts: Root, Leaves, Flowers, Fruits, Seeds & Seed oil.

Chemical constituents: Root contains Resin, Tannin, starch.

Seeds contain 50% oil, protein, Ricinine, Ricin, Lipase enzyme, Fixed oil.

Fixed oil contains Glycerides, Ricinolesis, Isoricinoleic acid, stearic acid, Crystals of calcium oxalate, nitrate.

Folk Use: Asthma, Headache, Rheumatism, Scorpion sting, Teething trouble

Use in literature: Fruits – Asthma, bronchitis, epilepsy, eye diseases, febrifuge, hydrocoel, jaundice, lumbago, piles, rheumatism, sciatica, skin diseases.

Leaves – Cough, worms infestation.

221. *Salvadora persica* L. Var. *wightiana* [Planch ex Thw.] Verdc. (Salvadoraceae)

Syn.: *S. indica* Wight.

Distribution: Rare.

Botany: A small or medium sized, crooked or bent. Leaves variable in shape ovate, elliptic-ovate or ovate lanceolate, pale Green, glossy, fleshy. Flowers Greenish-Yellow, in axillary & terminal panicles. Drupes globose, fleshy, dark Red at Maturity.

Flowering & Fruiting**:** December-March.

Medicinal Parts: Fruits.

Chemical Constituents: Root – Alkaloid-Trimethylamine, β-Sitosterol, Glucotropaeolin, Monoclinic Sulphur.

Stem- β-Sitosterol, Octacosanol, Salvadoside, Salvadoraside, Siringin.

Leaves – Salvadoricine.

Folk Use: Rheumatism

Use in literature: Leaves – Asthma, Bronchitis, Constipation, Cough, Haemorrhoids, Scurvy, Strangury, Verminosis.

Fruits – Constipation, Gastropathy, Seminal weakness.

222. *Schleichera oleosa* (Lour.) Oken. (Sapindaceae)

Syn.: *S. trijuga* Willd.

Vern.: Kusum.

Distribution: Common in dry deciduous forests, often along river banks. Bhopal, Hosahangabad, Mandla, Satna, Seoni, Shahdol.

Botany: A handsome tree. Leaves paripinnate. Flowers Yellowish-Green. Fruits pointed, Smooth or echinate. Flowering & Fruiting**:** March-August.

Medicinal Parts: Bark, Oil.

Chemical Constituents: Seed – Phenols, Polyene Pigments.

Seed oil – Cyanolipids, Oleic acid, Gadoleic acid, Stearic acid, Arachidic acid, Behenic acid, Palmitic acid, Palmitoleic acid.

Leaves – Stigmasterol, β-sitosterol, Campesterol, Cholesterol, Fructose, Glucose, Tartaric acid, Oxalic acid.

Folk Use: Rheumatism

Use in literature: Bark – Inflammation, Malaria, Pruritus, Ulcers.

Seed oil – Burns, Cephalalgia, Ulcers.

223. *Semecarpus anacardium* L. f. (Anacardiaceae)

Vern.: Bhelwa.

Distribution: Common in dry deciduous & Sal forests. Balaghat, Bhopal, Hosahangabad, Jabalpur, Mandla, Rewa, Seoni, Shahdol.

Botany: A small trees, with unisexual flowers and drupe fruits.

Flowering & Fruiting: May-March.

Medicinal Parts: Fruits.

Chemical Constituents: Fruits contain – Anacardiac acid, Cardol, Catechol, Anacardol, Fixed oil, Somearpol, Bhilawanol.

Folk Use: Asthma, Epilepsy, Psoriasis, Rheumatism

Use in literature: Fruits – Asthma, Caridac diseases, Colic, Constipation, Cough, Diabetes, Dyspepsia, Fever, Flatulence, General debility, Haemorrhoids, Helminthiasis, Hepatopathy, Sciatica, Scrofula, Tumours, Ulcers.

224. *Senna absus* (L.) Roxb. (Caesalpiniaceae)

Syn.: *Cassia absus* L.

Vern.: Chaksu.

Distribution: In waste lands. Balaghat, Bhopal, Damoh, E. Nimar, Indore, Mandla, Panna, Raisen, Sagar, Satna, Seoni, Shahdol, Shivpuri, Tikamgarh.

Botany: Annual herbs, clothed with glandular hairs; rachis grooved; leaflets obliquely elliptic to obovate; flowers pink or red, in terminal or leaf opposed, few-flowered racemes; pods hairy, flat.

Flowering & Fruiting: August –November.

Medicinal Parts: Leaves, seeds.

Chemical constituents: Seed contains Alkaloids, sugars, fats, cannins, mucilage, major protein, mangenese.

Folk Use: Ringworm, Sypilis, Wounds,

Use in literature: Leaf – Anaemia, asthma, cough, diarrhoea, hiccough, nasitis, tumours.

Seed – Diarrhoea, dysentery, haemorrhages, obesity, poisonous bites, ulcers, wounds.

225. *Senna occidentalis* (L.) Link. (Caesalpiniaceae)

Syn.: *Cassia occidentalis* L.

Vern.: Ban-chironta.

Distribution: In Wastelands. Bhopal, E. Nimar, Hosahangabad, Indore, Mandla, Panna, Raisen, Ratlam, Rewa, Sagar, Satna, Sidhi, Shivpuri, W. Nimar.

Botany: Diffuse undershrubs, with 3-6 pairs of leaflets and a gland on the petiole. Flowers yellow, in corymbose panicles. Pods linear-oblong.

Flowering & Fruiting: July-April.

Medicinal Parts: Leaves, Root.

Chemical constituents: Plant contains Emodin, Tannic acid, fatty oils, Mucilage, aminoacids, Chrysophanol, Sitosterol, Xanthon, Cassiodin, Nitrogen bases, Betain, Choline, Stachydrine, and Trigonelline.

Seed contains Galactomanon.

Folk Use: Asthma, Cough, Jaundice, Rheumatism

Use in literature: Root – Colic, diabetes, dyspepsia, elephantiasis, epilepsy, flatulence, inflammation, ringworm, scorpion sting.

Leaf – Asthma, bronchitis, cough, fever, hiccough, hydrophobia, leprosy, pruritus, ulcers, wounds.

Seed – Bronchitis, constipation, cough, dyspepsia, erysipelas, fever, flatulence, hiccough, leprosy, stranguray, ulcers.

226. *Shorea robusta* Gaertn. f. (Depterocarpaceae)

Vern.: Sal, Sarai.

Distribution: In well drained soil on lower hill slopes. Balaghat, Hosahangabad, Mandla, Rewa.

Botany: A large deciduous trees; flowers cream or Pale yellow, in racemes.

Flowering & Fruiting: March-June.

Medicinal Parts: Bark, leaves, resin & fruits.

Chemical constituents: Seed – Fatty oil.

Wood – Oleoresin.

Folk Use: Aphrodisiac, Deysentery, Gonorrhoea

Use in literature: Bark, Leaves, Seed – Anaemia, asthma, bleeding piles, cough, diabetes, diarrhoea, dysentery, ear diseases, fracture, gonorrhoea, leprosy, sprain, wounds.

Fruit – Burning sensation, seminal weakness, tubercular ulcers.

Resin – Burns, diarrhoea, dysentery, fever, gonorrhoea, pruritus, ulcers, wounds.

227. *Sida acuta* Burm. (Malvaceae)

Syn.: *S. carpinifolia* L. f.

Vern.: Mahabala.

Distribution: In wastelands, fallow fields, and along roadsides and forests. Balaghat, Damoh, Gwalior, Hosahangabad, Mandla, Raisen, Rewa, Sagar, Shivpuri, Sidhi.

Botany: Undershrubs; flowers Yellow, solitary axillary. Flowering & Fruiting: August-January.

Medicinal parts: Seed.

Chemical constituents:

Root contains – Alkaloids as β-Phenethylamine, Ephedrine, Vasicinol, Vasicinone, Vasicine, Choline, Hypaphorine, Betaine, Cryptolepine, Alpha-Amyrin.

Folk Use: Sexual vitality

Use in literature:

Root – Diabetes, Dysuria, Paralysis, Leucorrhoea, Nervous disorders, Sciatica, Tuberculosis, Urinary disorders.

228. *Sida cordata* Borsm. (Malvaceae)

Syn.: *S. humilis* Cav.; *S. veronicifolia* Lam.

Distribution: In Wastelands and forest margins. Balaghat, Bhopal, Damoh, Hosahangabad, Indore, Jabalpur, Mandla, Raisen, Rewa, Sagar, Satna, Seoni, Shivpuri, Sidhi.

Botany: Trailing hispid herbs, with solitary axillary Yellow flowers & schizocarpic fruits.

Flowering & Fruiting: Throughout the year.

Medicinal parts: Leaves, Root.

Chemical constituents: β-pheneethylamines; Quinazoline, Carboxylated tryptamine, Linoleic acid, Malavalic acid, Sterculic acid, Gossypol, Ephedrine, Vasicinol, Vasicinone, Vasicine, Choline, Betaine, Cholesterol, Stigmasterol.

Folk Use: Sexual vitality

Use in literature:

Root – Fever, Arthritis.

Root bark – Gonorrhoea, Leucorrhoea.

Leaves – Diarrhoea.

Flowers / Ripe fruits – Burning sensation.

229. *Sida cordifolia* L. (Malvaceae)

Vern.: Bala.

Distribution: In wastelands, forest margins and roadsides. Balaghat, Bhopal, Hosahangabad, Mandla, Seoni, Shivpuri, Sidhi.

Botany: Undershrubs, with ovate-cordate leaves and axillary yellow flowers. Mericarps 10, 2-awned.

Flowering & Fruiting: August– November.

Medicinal Parts: Root, leaves, seeds, whole plant.

Chemical constituents: Root contains Beta-sitosterol, alkaloids-visicinonoe, vasicine, vasicinol, choline, & betain.

Seeds contain Ephedrine, fatty oils, steroids, resin, mucin, sterculic acid, malvalic acid, linoleic acid, potassium nitrate.

Folk Use: Colic pain, Facial paralyseis, Sciatica, Sprematorrhoea, Leucorrhoea, Piles

Use in literature: Plant – Cough.

Bark – Urinary trouble & discharges.

Fruits – Blood diseases, diseases of throat, piles.

230. *Sida rhombifolia* L. (Malvaceae)

Vern.: Atibala.

Distribution: In wastelands, rock-crevices, forests and along streams. Balaghat, Bhopal, Hosahangabad, Mandla, Seoni, Shivpuri, Sidhi.

Botany: Much-branched herbs, with obovate- rounded or rhomboid leaves and axillary, solitary, yellow flowers. Mericarps 1-awned or awnless.

Flowering & Fruiting: October – December.

Medicinal Parts: Whole plant, root, leaves.

Chemical constituents: Plant contains Ephedrine, cellulose, lignin, quanozolines, β- Phenethylamines, Tryptomine, Sterculic acid, Malvalic acid, Linoleic acid.

Folk Use: Leucorrhoea, Rheumatism, Tuberculosis

Use in literature: Root – Burning sensation, fever, heart diseases, inflammation, Piles, strangury, urinary complaints.

Leaf – Burning sensation, fever, heart diseases, inflammation, Piles, strangury, urinary complaints.

231. *Solanum nigrum* L. (Solanaceae)

Syn.: *S. subrum* Mill. Ex Wight.; *S. incertum* Dunal ex Grahum.

Vern.: Makoi.

Distribution: In wastelands and moist places throughout the State. Chhatarpur, Damoh, Hosahangabad.

Botany: Unarmed, glabrous or pubescent herbs, with ovate-oblong leaves, white flowers and globose, yellow, red or purple fruits.

Flowering & Fruiting: September– February.

Medicinal Parts: Whole plant, flowers, leaves, fruits.

Chemical constituents: Plant contains Alkaloids, Reducing sugars, glycosides, saponins, steroids, leutein, Lycopene, Vitamin – C, glucose, fructose, caffeic – solasodine, tomatidenel, solamargine, solasomine, trigogenine, potassium, Iron, sulphur, Calcium, Phosphorus.

Folk Use: Jaundice, Snake bite

Use in literature: Fruits – Asthma, bronchitis, cough, dysentery, erysipelas, eye diseases, fever, heart diseases, hiccough, inflammation, itching, leucoderma, piles, urinary discharges, vomiting, worms in the ear.

232. *Solanum surattense* Burm. f. (Solanaceae)

Syn.: *S. maccanni* Sant.; *S. xanthocarpum* Schrad. & Wendl.; *S. diffusum* Roxb.; *S. armatum* Br.; *S. virginianum* Jacq.

Vern.: Bhuri rindi.

Distribution: In open wastelands throughout the State. Balaghat, Chhatarpur, Damoh, Dhar, E. Nimar, Hosahangabad, Indore, Mandla, Panna, Rewa, Satna, Seoni, Sidhi, Tikamgarh; W. Nimar.

Botany: Prostrate, prickly herbs, with sinuately lobed to subpinnatifid leaves. Flowers violet-purple or white. Fruits globose, yellow when ripe.

Flowering & Fruiting: December-June.

Medicinal Parts: Whole plant, fruits, seeds.

Chemical constituents: Plant contains Alkaloids (Solasonine), diosgenin. Solacinine.

Seed contains Essential oil, solanocarpine.

Flower contains Flavonol, glycoside, queretin, apigenin, sitosterol.

Leaves contain Coumarine, scopolin, esculin, esculetin.

Folk Use: Asthma, Cough, Rheumatisms

Use in literature: Root – Asthma, bronchitis, fever, heart diseases, lumbago, pains, piles, strangury.

Fruits – Asthma, fever, heart diseases, pruritus.

233. *Soymida febrifuga* A. Juss. (Meliaceae)

Syn.: *Swietenia febrifuga* Roxb.

Vern.: Rohan.

Distribution: Jabalpur.

Botany: A tall glabrous deciduous trees; flowers Greenish-White, in terminal or axillary panicles.

Flowering & Fruiting: March-May.

Medicinal Parts: Bark.

Chemical constituents: Bark contains Bitter resinous substance, tannic acid, galic acid.

Folk Use: Rheumatism

Use in literature: Chronic fever, diarrhoea, dysentery, malaria fever, skin diseases, throat diseases, wounds.

234. *Sphaeranthus indicus* L. (Asteraceae)

Syn.: *S. hirtus* Willd

Distribution: Common in dry open forests. Balaghat, Damoh, Hosahangabad.

Botany – Prostrate or decumbent-ascending, aromatic annual herb with Purple flowers & Achenes fruits. Flowering & Fruiting: November-March.

Medicinal parts – Leaves, Floral bud.

Chemical constituents: Essential oil contains – Methyl Chavicol, α-Ionone, d-Cadinene, p-Methoxycinnamaldehyde, α-Terpinene, Citral, Geraniol, Geranyl acetate, β-Ionane, Sphaerene, Indicusene, Sphaeranthol.

Folk Use: Cojunctivitis, Earache

Use in literature: Flowers – Conjunctivitis, Skin diseases.

Root & Seed – Intestinal worms, Indigestion, Cough.

235. *Strychnos potatorum* L. f. (Loganiaceae)

Vern.: Kaya.

Distribution: In mixed forests. Hosahangabad, Seoni.

Distribution: West Bengal, Central & South India upto 1,200 m.

Botany: Medium sized deciduous glabrous trees, with fragrant White flowers & berries fruits. Flowering & Fruiting: April-July.

Medicinal Parts: Leaves, Stem bark.

Chemical Constituents: Seeds – Brucine, Diaboline, β-Sitosterol, Stigmasterol, Oleanolic acid and its 3B-acetate and a Saponin, Galactose and Mannose from Seeds.

Leaf & Bark – Isomotiol, Mixture of Sitosterol, Stigmasterol, Campsterol.

Folk Use: Cholera, Ulcer

Use in literature: Seed – Bronchitis, Burning sensation, Chronic diarrhoea, Conjunctivitis, Diabetes, Dipsia, Dysentery, Gastropathy, Gonorrhoea, Leucorrhoea, Strangury, Ulcers.

Root – Leprosy.

236. *Syzygium cumini* (L.) Skeels (Myrtaceae)

Syn.: *Eugenia jambolana* Lam.

Vern.: Jamun.

Distribution: Growing in sal forest margins, along road sides, streams and rivers. Balaghat, Damoh, Hosahangabad, Mandla, Shahdol, Shivpuri, Sidhi.

Botany: Trees, with elliptic-lanceolate leaves and pale-green or white flowers in axillary paniculate cymes. Fruits globose or oblong, purple when ripe.

Flowering & Fruiting: February-August.

Medicinal Parts: Leaves, bark, fruits, seed.

Chemical constituents: Bark contains Friedelin, kaempferol, tannins, quercetin, β- sitosterol, betullinic acid.

Fruits contains Anthocyanin, eugin.

Seed contains Ellagic acid, IAA, Oxalic acid, citric acid, glycollic acid, glucose, fructose, gallic acid.

Leaves contain Glycine, alanin, leucin, tyrosin.

Folk Use: Diabetes, Diarrhoea, Diuretic, Dysentery, Dyspepsia

Use in literature: Bark – Asthma, biliousness, blood diseases, bronchitis, dysentery, Sore throat, ulcer.

Fruits – Biliousness.

Seed – Diabetes.

237. *Tamarindus indica* L. (Caesalpiniaceae)

Syn.: *T. officinalis* Hook.; *T. occidentalis* Gaertn.

Vern.: Imli.

Distribution: Balaghat, Bhopal, Damoh, Indore, Jabalpur, Mandla, Raisen, Shahdol, Shivpuri, Sidhi.

Botany: Evergreen trees, with 6-12 pairs of leaflets and yellow with purple streaks. Pods subtorulose, falcate.

Flowering & Fruiting: May-August.

Medicinal Parts: Fruits, seeds.

Chemical constituents: Polysaccharides, balsamine, catechin, nasturtium, tamarin, phosphatidic acid and its choline, ethanollamine, serine, inositol, alkaloid, citric acid, tartaric acid, potassium bitartrate.

Folk Use: Scorpion sting, Snake bite, Sunstoke

Use in literature: Bark – Gonorrhoea, paralysis, urinary discharges.

Leaf – Blood diseases, earaehe, eye diseases, inflammation, ophthamia, ringworm, small pox, snake bite, swelling, tumor.

Flower – Urinary discharges.

Fruits – Wound fractures.

Seed – Ulcers, vaginal discharges.

238 Tectona grandis L. f. (Verbenaceae)

Vern.: Sagwan.

Distribution Balaghat, Chhatarpur, Dhar, Hosahangabad, Panna, Rewa, Seoni, Tikamgarh.

Botany: Deciduous trees, with broadly elliptic large leaves. Flowers white or pinkish, stamens all equal. Fruits enclosed in bladder-like inflated calyx.

Flowering & Fruiting: September–December.

Medicinal Parts: Bark.

Chemical constituents: Tactograndon, Betulin, Lupeol, Betulinic acid, Betulinaldehyde, Carbohydrates, fatty acids, lapachanone, deoxylapachol, tectoquinine.

Folk Use: Snake bite

Use in literature:

Flower – Biliousness, bronchitis, urinary discharges.

Bark – Bronchitis.

Wood – Biliousness, dysentery, leucoderma, piles.

239. *Tephrosia purpurea* Pers. (Papilionaceae)

Syn.: *T. villosa* Pers.; *T. maxima* Pers.; *T. lanceolata* R. Grah., *T. hamiltonaii* Drumm ex Gamble.

Vern.: Sarphonka.

Distribution: Balaghat, Bhopal, Bhind, Dhar, Hosahangabad, Indore, Jabalpur, Mandla, Morena, Narsimhapur, Panna, Raisen, Rewa, Sagar, Satna, Seoni, Shahdol, Shivpuri, Sidhi, Tikamgarh.

Botany: Perennial, woody herbs, with 11-21 leaflets and reddish-purple or bright pink to white flowers in leaf-opposed racemes. Style glabrous.Pods linear.

Flowering & Fruiting: Throughout the year.

Medicinal Parts: Leaves, Root.

Chemical constituents: Beta-Sitosterol, Cyanidin Chloride, Pongomol, Lupeol, Rutin, Dephinindinchloride, Karangin, Kangone, flevichapparins – B and C, Methylkaranjic acid, Purgurin.

Root contains Tephrosin, Degulin, Rotenone, Isotephrosin, alterative.

Folk Use: Asthma, Diarrhoea, Dysentery, Fever, Rheumatism, Stiffness, Tonsilitis

Use in literature: Diseases of blood, heart, liver, spleen. asthma, bronchitis, leprosy, snake bite, tumour, ulcer, wound.

240. *Teramnus labialis* (L. f.) Spr. (Papilionaceae)

Vern.: Mashoni.

Distribution: Climbing on roadsides bushes. Balaghat, Damoh, Gwalior, Hosahangabad, Indore, Jabalpur, Mandla, Narsimhapur, Panna, Raisen, Rewa, Sagar, Seoni, Shahdol, Shivpuri, Sidhi.

Botany: A climbing wide spreading hairy herb; leaves trifoliate, leaflets are of unequal size; flowers pink or bluish white.

Flowering & Fruiting: August-April.

Medicinal Parts: Leaves, Fruits, Seeds.

Chemical constituents: Galactomannan, carbohydrates, sugars, amino acids, fatty acids, carotene, saponins, sapogenin, diosgenin, gitogenin, neogitogenin; Alkaloids, Saponeritin, neogigenin, tigogecnin, vicenin, vitexin, luteolin, yamogenin, furastanolglycosides, kaempfrol, quercetin.

Folk Use: Rheumatism

Use in literature: Seeds – Anaemia, colic, cough, diabetes, diarrhoea, dropsy, dysentery, rheumatism, rickets.

241. *Terminalia arjuna* (Roxb.) Wt. & Arn. (Combretaceae)

Vern.: Arjun,

Distribution: Along banks of streams and rivers, and in mixed forests. Balaghat, Bhopal, Chhatarpur, Chhindwara, Damoh, Hosahangabad, Indore, Jabalpur, Mandla, Raisen, Rewa, Sagar, Satna, Seoni, Shahdol, Shivpuri, Sidhi, Tikamgarh.

Botany: Trees, with smooth bark and leaves cordate at base. Flowers white, in axillary spikes or terminal panicles. Fruits 5-winged, wings curved upwards.

Flowering: April-May.

Fruiting: Almost throughout the year.

Medicinal Parts: Bark, leaves.

Chemical constituents: Bark contains Bita- sitosterol, Arjunic acid, Friedlene, Glucoside, (Arjunetic), Tannins, Sugars, Sodium, Magnessium, Aluminium, Calcium Carbonate.

Folk Use: Dysentery, Heart tonic, Menorrhoea

Use in literature: Bark – Asthma, biliousness, blood diseases, fractures, leucoderma, tumour, ulcer, urinary discharges.

242. *Terminalia bellerica* (Gaentn.) Roxb. (Combretaceae)

Vern.: Bahera.

Distribution: In mixed and Sal forests. Balaghat, Bhopal, Damoh Hosahangabad, Indore, Jabalpur, Mandla, Raisen, Rewa, Sagar, Satna, Seoni, Shahdol, Shivpuri, Sidhi.

Botany: Deciduous trees, with broadly obovate leaves clustered at the end of branches. Flowers yellow or creamy white, in spikes. Fruits ellipsoid, 5-ridged.

Flowering: April-May.

Fruiting: Most part of the year.

Medicinal Parts: Fruits, Seed oil.

Chemical constituents: Fruits contain β- Sitosterol, gallic acid, ellagic acid, Chebulagic acid, Galloyl, Glucose, Many free sugars, Manitol, galactose, Rhamnose, glucoside.

Folk Use: Diarrhoea, Dropsy, Dyspepsia, Rheumatism

Use in literature: Bark- Anaemia, leucoderma

Fruits – Asthma, biliousness, bronchitis, cardiac diseases, inflammation, sore throat.

243. *Terminellia chebula* (Gaentn.) Retz. (Combretaceae)

Vern.: Harra

Distribution: In dry deciduous and sal forests. Balaghat, Betul, Chhindwada, Damoh, Hosahangabad, Indore, Jabalpur, Mandla, Raisen, Seoni, Shahdol, Sidhi.

Botany: Deciduous trees, Leaves ovate or elliptic. Flowers Yellow or creamy white, in spikes. Fruits 5-ridged.

Flowering: April June.

Fruiting: Winter Season.

Medicinal Parts: Galls.

Chemical constituents: Fruits contain- Tannic acid, gallic acid, chebulinic acid, mucilage, glycoside (Anthroquinine), Carbohydrates, amino acids, phosphoric acid, succinic acid.

Folk Use: Asthma.

Use in literature: Fruits – Anaemia, ascities, asthma, biliousness, constipation, elephantiasis, gout, hiccough, inflammation, leucoderma, piles, sore throat, strangury, tumour, typhoid, urinary discharges, vesicular calculi, vomiting.

244. *Thespesia populnea* (L.) Soland. ex Correa. (Malvaceae)

Syn.: *Hibiscus populnea* L.

Distribution: Commonly planted as an avenue tree. Bhopal, Dhar.

Botany: Small evergreen trees, with yellow flowers and brown capsule fruits.

Flowering & Fruiting: September-August.

Medicinal Parts: Bark, stem, leaves, root, fruit.

Chemical constituents: Leaves contain Lupeol, lupenone, B-sitosterol.

Stem contains Calycopterin, sequiterpenoid quinones.

Fruits contains Thespesin, gossypol, populinin, populneol, herbacetin, populnetin, gossypectin, epoxyleic acid, isoquercitrin, rutin, B-sitosterol, thespesone.

Folk Use: Jaundice, Hair loss.

Use in literature: Bark – Cough, diabetes, dysentery, dyspepsia, gonorrhoea, headache, itching, influenza, indigestion, psoriasis, typhoid, ulcers.

Leaves – Cough, eczema, fever, headache, inflammations, influenza, psoriasis, scabies.

Root – Inflammations, psoriasis, scabies.

Fruit – Cancer, eczema, malaria, migrain, scabies, psoriasis, ringworm, tumours.

245. *Thevetia peruviana* (Pers.) Schum. (Apocynaceae)

Syn.: *T. nerifolia* Juss. ex Steud.; *Cascabela thevetia* (L.) Lipp.

Vern.: Pili kaner.

Distribution: Cultivated in gardens and parks. Balaghat, Chhatarpur, Damoh, Indore, Panna, Sidhi.

Botany: A large evergreen shrub or small trees, with linear leaves, yellow flowers and subglobose fruits.

Flowering & Fruiting: Throughout the year.

Medicinal Parts: Seeds.

Chemical constituents: Seeds contain – Theveside, viridoside, thevefolin, thevetin, thevetoxin, peruvoside, ruvoside.

Flowers & Fruits contain – Epiperuviol acetate, α – & β – amyrin, kaempferol, quercetin, glycoside- thevetin & other thevetoxin.

Folk Use: Rheumatism

Use in literature: Bark – Dropsy, oedema, rheumatism.

246. *Tinospora cordifolia* (Willd.) Miers. ex Hk. f. & Th. (Menispermaceae)

Syn.: *T. glabra* (N. Burm.) Merr.; *Cocculus cordifolius* DC.; *Menispermum cordifolium* Willd.

Vern.: Gurcha.

Distribution: On tree in the forests. Bhopal, Indore, Rewa, Sagar, Satna.

Botany: Succulent, glabrous, deciduous climbers, with corky and lenticelled bark. Leaves ovate-cordate. Flowers yellow, in axillary racemes. Fruits globose, red when ripe.

Flowering & Fruiting: August-February.

Medicinal Parts: Whole plant, Stem, Juice of fresh plant, Fruit.

Chemical constituents: Starch, Glycoside (Giloin), Tinosporic acid, Vasa alcohol, essential oil, Vasa acid, Proteins, Calcium, Phosphorus, Berberine, gilosterol.

Folk Use: Debility, Diabetes, Fever, Jaundice, Leprosy, Rheumatism, Sleeplessness, Snake bite, Stone trouble, Sunstoke, Vomiting

Use in literature: Stem – Burning sensation, constipation, diabetes, enriches the blood, fevers, Jaundice, skin diseases, spleen diseases tonic, vaginal discharges, vomiting.

247. *Trachyspermum ammi* (L.) Spragae. (Apiaceae)

Syn.: *Carum copticum* Benth & Hook.

Vern.: Ajwain.

Distribution: Cultivated. Damoh, Hosahangabad.

Botany: Annual herbs, with whitish or pinkish flowers and muricated fruits. Flowering & Fruiting: November-March.

Medicinal Parts: Fruits, Leaves, Seed Oil.

Chemical Constituents: Fruits contain – An aromatic Volatile oil, Stearoptene, Cumene, Terpene as Thymine; Phenolic Glucosides; Thymol, p-cymene, Stearoptin, Cymon, Terpene.

Folk Use: Cold, Dyspepsia, Pneumonia

Use in literature: Fruits – Abdominal Colic & Pain, Cholera, Diarrhoea, Dyspepsia, Flatulence, Heart tonic, Helminthiasis, Indigestion, Rheumatism, Uritcaria.

Leaves – Abdominal pain, Cholera, Colic, Diarrhoea, Flatulence, Heart diseases, Helminthiasis, Indigestion, Rheumatism, Urticaria.

248. *Trianthema portulacastrum* L. (Azoiaceae)

Distribution: Common on railway tracts and roadsides.

Botany: Succulent, prostrate herbs, with spathulate leaves. Flowers white or pink, solitary; stamens 10. capsules mitrifrom.

Flowering & Fruiting: August.

Medicinal Parts: Roots, Leaves, Fruits, Seeds.

Chemical Constituents: Protein, fat, carbohydrate, crude fibre, calcium, phosphorus, Iron, ascorbic acid, carotene, oxalates.

Folk Use: Jaundice, Leucorrhoea, Urinary trouble

Use in literature: Plant – Anaemia, Ascites, Bronchitis, Heart diseases of the blood, Inflammation, Piles,

Root – Night blindness.

249. *Tribulus terrestris* L. (Zygophyllaceae)

Vern.: Gokhru.

Distribution: Hosahangabad, Indore, Ratlam, Satna, Sidhi, Tikamgarh.

Botany: Procumbent annual herbs, with pinnate leaves and yellow flowers. Mericarps dorsally tuberculate, spines 4.

Flowering & Fruiting: May-June.

Medicinal Parts: Fruits, roots, Whole plant.

Chemical constituents: Fruits contains Alkaloid, fixed oil, essential oil, Resin, Steroids, Saponins, Vitamin- C, Protein, Nitrates.

Folk Use: Gout, Kideny trouble, Leucorrhoea, Rheumatism, Urinary complaints.

Use in literature: Root – Asthma, blood diseases, burning sensation, cough, inflammation, pruritus, strangury urinary discharges, vesicular calculi.

Fruits – Asthma, blood diseases, burning sensation, cough, inflammation, pruritus, strangury urinary discharges, vesicular calculi.

Seed **–** Inflammation, stones in bladder, urinary trouble.

250 *Trichodesma indicum* (L.) R. Br. (Boraginaceae)

Vern.: Chhota-Kulpha.

Distribution: Common in wastelands, grassy fields & along roadsides. Dhar, Indore, Seoni.

Botany: An erect or diffuse, much branched, Grey-Villous hispid herb. Leaves mostly sessile lanceolate or cordate-lanceolate. Flowers pale-Blue or Violet or White with Brown throat. Nutlets rough on the inner face, obscurely margined.

Flowering & Fruiting: July-November.

Medicinal Parts: Root.

Folk Use- Rheumatism

Use in literature: Plant – Diarrhoea, Dysentery, Dysmenorrhoea, Dyspepsia, Fever, Inflammation, Leprosy, Skin diseases, Strangury,

251. *Tridax procumbens* L. (Asteraceae)

Distribution: Common in waste moist places. Balaghat, Hosahangabad, Satna.

Botany: Straggling herbs, with ovate-lanceolate leaves & yellow heads terminating long peduncles. Achenes silky.

Flowering & Fruiting: Throughout the year.

Medicinal Parts: Leaves, Whole plant.

Chemical Constituents: Leaf – Fumaric acid.

Flowers – Glucoluteolin, Luteolin, Isoquercetin, Quercetin.

Folk Use: Cuts, Piles, Wounds,

Use in literature: Wounds, Boils.

252. *Trigonella foenum-graceum* L. (Papilionaceae)

Vern.: Methi.

Distribution: Cultivated for seeds, used as a spice. Bhopal, Shivpuri.

Botany: An aromatic, erect, annual herbs with 3-foliate leaves and pale yellow flowers in axils of young leaves; pods 8-10 cm. long, with long beak.

Flowering & Fruiting**:** February.

Medicinal Parts: Leaves, Seeds.

Chemical constituents: Seed contains – Quercetin, luteolin, trigonelline, choline, nicotinic acid, fixed oil, essential oil, mucilage, bitter extractive, colouring matter, 2 steroidal saponins.

Folk Use: Rheumatism

Use in literature: Seeds – Bronchitis, cough, dropsy, epilepsy, fever, gout, paralysis, vomiting.

253. *Triumfetta rhomboidea* Jacq. (Tiliaceae)

Syn.: *T. bartramia* L.; *T. angulata* Lam.

Distribution: Along the forest margins & roadsides. Hosahangabad, Jabalpur, Mandla, Sagar, Seoni, Shahdol, Sidhi.

Botany: Stout herbs, with ovate-rounded, 3-lobed & entire Leaves. Flowers yellow, with 5-10 stamens. Capsules pubescent, spines glabrous.

Flowering & Fruiting**:** August-November.

Medicinal Parts: Leaves, Root.

Chemical Constituents: Plant contains – 4-Hydroxyisoxazole and Triumboidin.

Folk Use: Boils, Proleps of uterus, Urinogenital diseases of men.

Use in literature: Root – Dysentery.

254. *Typha elephantina* Roxb. (Typhaceae)

Syn.: *T. angustifolia* Watt. Non L.

Vern.: Aer.

Distribution: Common & gregarious in marshy & water logged places along roadsides and in ditches throughout the state.

Botany: Erect, rhizomatous herbs, with spongy linear leaves flat above and convex beneath. Spikes cylindrical, male flowers above, female below and up to 3 cm long gap in between. Flowering & Fruiting: Throughout the year.

Medicinal Parts: Down of Fruit.

Chemical Constituents: Seed yield a fatty oil.

Folk Use: Antiseptic, Cuts, Wounds

Use in literature: Whole plant – Burning sensation, Gonorrhoea, Inflammation, Leprosy, Splenic enlargement, Strangury.

255. *Uraria picta* Desv. (Papilionaceae)

Syn.: *Hedysarum pictum* Jacq.

Vern.: Dabra, Pithwan.

Distribution: Growing as undergrowth of forest. Balaghat, Damoh, Hosahangabad, Mandla, Raisen, Sagar, Satna, Seoni, Shahdol, Sidhi.

Botany: An erect, little-branched perennial undershurbs; upper leaflets white-clouded; flowers purple; pods white or greyish, polished.

Flowering & Fruiting: August-January.

Medicinal Parts: Root, Fruit.

Chemical constituents: 5-hydroxy-7, 4-dimithoxy flavonol & 5 other flavonoids.

Folk Use: Fever, Mouth sores, Piles, Snake bite

Use in literature: Bleeding piles, burning sensation, cough, diarrhoea, intermittent fever, rheumatism, ulcer.

256. *Urginea indica* (Roxb.) Kunth. (Liliaceae)

Syn.: *Drimia indica* (Roxb.) Jessop.

Vern.: Jangli kanda/Jangli piyaz.

Distribution: In open dry situations, sometimes amongst stones and gravels in open places or shades. Rewa, Satna.

Botany: A small geophyte with ovoid, tunicated, white bulb, leaves radical, linear-lanceolate; flowers pale-brown, on a leafless scape, in few flowered racemes; capsule long, ellipsoid; seeds elliptic, black.

Flowering & Fruiting: March-May.

Medicinal Parts: Bulbs.

Chemical constituents: Bulb contain Glucosides, Scillian, Scillipicrin, Scillitin, Mucilage, Sugars, Calcium oxalate.

Folk Use: Cholera, Cough, Rheumatic pain, Snake bite

Use in literature: Asthma, blood pressure, cough, menorrhagia, paralysis, pneumonia fever, skin diseases, whooping cough.

257. *Vernonia cinerea* (L.) Less (Asteraceae)

Syn.: *Conyza cinerea* L.

Vern.: Sahadevi.

Distribution: Very common throughout the State, on roadsides and in waste places.

Botany: Erect or decumbent herbs, with ovate to obovate or variable leaves. Heads violet or pink. Achenes terete.

Flowering & Fruiting: Throughout the year.

Medicinal Parts: Root, flower, seeds, whole plant.

Chemical constituents: Plant contains Lupeol acetate, alpha – amyrin, acetate, glucoside, Quercetin, β- sitosterol, stigma sterol, œ-spina sterol, potassium chhoride, œ- amyrin, lupeol.

Flower contains Luteolin, Iso – orientin, chrysoeriol.

Folk Use: Piles, Rheumatism

Use in literature: Plant – Asthma, bronchitis.

258. *Vetiveria zizanioides* (L.) Nash. (Poaceae)

Syn.: *Andropogon muricatus* Retz.

Vern.: Khas-khas.

Distribution: Balaghat, Damoh, Gwalior, Hosahangabad, Rewa, Sagar.

Botany: A densely tufted, erect perennial aromatic grasses; sessile spikelets awnless; yellow scabrous when mature.

Flowering & Fruiting: August-November.

Medicinal Parts: Roots, Root oil.

Chemical constituents: Root contains – Essential oil, resin, acidic substance, iron, calcium, salts, citronellal, geraniol, terpene, Lignin.

Folk Use: Menstrual disorders, Rheumatism

Use in literature: Roots – Anaemia, asthma, burning sensation, colic, dyspepsia, fever, hiccough, leprosy, menorrhagia, skin diseases, ulcers, vomiting.

259. *Vitex negundo* L. (Verbenaceae)

Vern.: Negur.

Distribution: Common along roadsides, river bank and cultivated fields. Balaghat, Betul, Chhatarpur, Damoh, Hosahangabad, Indore, Jabalpur, Mandla, Panna, Sagar, Satna, Seoni, Shivpuri, Sidhi, Tikamgarh.

Botany: Evergreen shrubs, with 3 to 5-foliolate leaves. Flowers violet, in peduncled cymes. Fruits ovoid, 4-celled.

Flowering & Fruiting: June-December.

Medicinal Parts: Leaves, flowers.

Chemical constituents: Volatile oil, Alkaloids (Nergundin & Hydrocotylon), Vitamin- C, Carotene, flavon, Tannic acid, Hydroxy benzoic acid, Resin, Mallic acid.

Folk Use: Cardiac trouble, Liver diseases, Rheumatism

Use in literature: Asthma, biliousness, bronchitis, enlargement of the spleen, eye diseases, inflammation, leucoderma.

260. *Withania somnifera* (L.) Dunal (Solanaceae)

Vern.: Ashwagandha.

Distribution: In wastelands.

Botany: Hoary-tomentose undershrubs, with elliptic-lanceolate or obovate leaves, bisexual flowers and berries enclosed in the persistent calyx.

Flowering & Fruiting: August- December.

Medicinal Parts: Root.

Chemical constituents: Root contains Alkaloids (Somniferon), Withaminon, Wasamin, Sugars, Glycosides, Amino acids, essential oils, Withaniol, Hentriacontane, Phytosterol & Oils.

Leaves contain Withanoloids alkaloids, glycosoids, glucose, amina acids.

Stem contains Proteins, amino acids, Tannin, flavonoids, Calcium, Iron.

Folk Use: Diuretic, Paralysis, Rheumatism, Tonic, Tuberculosis

Use in literature: Tuber – Asthma, bronchitis, inflammation, insomnia, psoriasis, scabies, ulcers.

261. *Wrightia tinctoria* (Roxb.) R. Br. (Apocynaceae)

Syn.: *W. rothii* G. Don.; *Nerium tinctorium* Roxb.

Vern.: Indrajau.

Distribution: Rare. Hoshangabad.

Botany: A small tree with glabrous young parts; leaves elliptic-oblong; flowers in lax, terminal corymbose, dichotomous cymes. Fruits follicles. Seeds with a tuft of hairs at the base.

Flowering & Fruiting: March-October.

Medicinal Parts: Stem Bark.

Chemical constituents: Seed contains – Fixed oil.

Bark – β-sitosterol, β-amyrin, lupeol benzoate.

Folk Use: Dysentery, Stomachache

Use in literature: Bark & Seeds – Burning sensation, colic, diarhroea, dropsy, dysentery, fever, flatulence, helminthiasis, leprosy, psoriasis.

Leaves – Hypertension.

262. *Xanthium strumarium* L. (Asteraceae)

Syn.: *X. indicum* Koenig ex Roxb.

Vern.: Adhasisi.

Distribution: Throghout the State as an Weed.

Botany: Foetid-smelling unarmed herbs, about 1m high. Leaves ovate-suborbicular. Heads greenish yellow, in terminal and axillary racemes.

Flowering & Fruiting: January – February.

Medicinal Parts: Root.

Chemical constituents:

Seed contains Xanthostrumarin acid, oxalic acid.

Fruits contain Strumaroside, stigmasterol, xanathin, xanthinin, xanthumin, xanthanol.

Folk Use: Migrain, Tonic

Use in literature: biliousness, epilepsy, fever, leucoderma, salivation.

263. *Zingiber officinale* Rosc. (Zingiberaceae)

Vern.: Adrak.

Distribution: Cultivated. Bhopal, Chhatarpur, Indore.

Botany: A small herb with horizontal, fleshy rhizome; leaves distichous, narrow, oblong-lanceolate; Flowers on long spike and are of purple colour on spike, small.

Flowering & Fruiting: September-October.

Medicinal Parts: Rhizome.

Chemical constituents: Rhizome contains Essential oil, Fibres, Proteins, Starch, Carbohydrates, Resin, Glutamin, Thrionin, Free amino acids, Zingiberol, Zingiberin, Glutamic acid, Aspartic acid.

Folk Use: Asthma, Cough, Gastric trouble

Use in literature: Rhizome – Arthritis, asthma, chronic bronchitis, cold, cough, dysuria, flatulence, gout, joint problems, lumbago, muscular trouble, rheumatism, sciatica, slip disc.

264. *Ziziphus mauritiana* Lam. (Rhamnaceae)

Syn.: *Z. jujuba* Mill.; *Z. vulgaris* Lam.; *Z. sativa* Gaertn.

Vern.: Ber.

Distribution Balaghat, Damoh, Hosahangabad, Indore, Mandla, Panna, Sagar, Satna, Shivpuri, Sidhi.

Botany: Evergreen small trees or shrubs, with droopling branches armed with prickles. Leaves ovate-elliptic to suborbicular, tomentose beneath. Flowers greenish- yellow, in axillary cllusters. Drupes fleshy.

Flowering & Fruiting: September-June.

Medicinal Parts: Bark, fruits.

Chemical constituents: Fruits contains Sugars & mucilage.

Folk Use: Dysentery

Use in literature: Root – Biliousness, headache.

Bark – Boils, diarrhoea, dysentery.

Leaf – Biliousness, diarrhoea, obesity.

Fruits – Biliousness, blood diseases, vomiting.

Seed – Asthma, burning sensation, cough, eye diseases, leucorrhoea, vomiting.

265. *Ziziphus nummularia* (Burm. F.) Wt. & Arn. (Rhamnaceae)

Syn.: *Z. rotundifolia* Lam.; *Rhamnus nummularia* Burm f.

Vern.: Jharberi.

Distribution: Hosahangabad, Shivpuri, Sidhi.

Botany: Much-branched, prickly shrubs, with zigzag branches & orbicular-ovate leaves tomentose above. Flowers greenish-yellow, in axillary cymes. Drupes globose, red when ripe. Flowering & Fruiting: **September-October.**

Medicinal Parts: Root, Fruits.

Chemical Constituents: Twig bark contains Tannin.

Root bark contains Cyclopeptide alkaloids Nummularine A, B, C; Mucronine-D & Amphibine-H.

Fol Uses: Blood purifier, Dysentery

Use in literature: Leaves – Cold, coughs, Scabies, Skin diseases.

Fruits – Bilious affections.

266. *Ziziphus oenoplia* (L.) Mill. (Rhamnaceae)

Vern.: Makoya.

Distribution: Balaghat, Bhopal, Damoh, Gwalior, Hosahangabad, Panna, Raisen, Rewa, Sagar, Satna, Seoni, Shahdol, Shivpuri, Sidhi.

Botany: A straggling or climbing shrub. Prickles paired one straight the other recurved. Leaves ovate, pointed; base oblique. Flowers in short axillary, dichotomous cymes. Drupes globose or obovoid, Black, shining. Flowering & Fruiting: May-October.

Medicinal Parts: Fruit.

Chemical Constituents: Bark contain tannin.

Stem & Root bark contain Cyclopeptide alkaloids Zizyphine-A & Zizyphine-B.

Folk Use: Burning sensation during urination, Dysentery

Use in literature: Roots – Ascaris Infection, Hyperacidity, Stomachalgia, Wounds.

Glossary of Medical Terms

Abortifacient	: an agent that induces abortion
Acrid	: biting, pungent
Adenitis	: inflammation of a gland or group of glands (or glandlike structures)
Agalactia	: absence or failure of secretion of milk
Alexipharmic	: antidote to poison
Alexiteric	: protective to infectious diseases
Alopecia	: loss of hair: a malady in which the hair falls from one or more circumscribed round or oval areas, leaving the skin smooth and white
Alterative	: causing a favourable change in the disordered functions of the body or metabolism
Amenorrhoea	: failure of menstruation
Amentia	: an arrest of the development of the mind from birth to early age
Anaemia	: lack of enough blood causing paleness
Analgesic	: an anodyne
Anaphrodisiac	: having the power to lessen or inhibit sexual feeling
Anodyne	: a medicine that allays pain
Anorexia	: a condition of having lost the appetite for food
Anthelmintic	: destroying or expelling worms
Antibacterial	: active against bacteria
Antidote	: an agent which neutralises or opposes the action of a poison
Anti-inflammatory	: acting against inflammation
Anti-leprotic	: any agent which prevents or cures leprosy
Antilithic	: an agent which prevents the formation of calculi
Anti-periodic	: preventing the regular recurrence of a disease
Antipyretic	: counteracting fever
Antiscorbutic	: acting against scurvy
Anti-septic	: a chemical sterilising substance to kill or control pathogenic microbes

Antispasmodic	:	opposing Spasms
Anuria	:	failure of the kidneys to produce urine
Aperient	:	A laxative
Aphrodisiac	:	drug which stimulates sexual desire
Areata	:	ocurring in circumscribed areas or patches
Arthritis	:	inflammation of joints
Ascities	:	an abnormal accumulation of a fluid in the peritoneal cavity
Astringent	:	a drug which contracts the organic tissues & canals of the body, & therby checking or deminishing bleeding of excessive discharges
Azoospermia	:	the comlete absence of sperm from the seminal fluid
Baldness	:	absence of hair from areas where it normally grows
Beriberi	:	a deficiency disease caused by imbalance of carbohydrate and vitamin B
Biliousness	:	a symptom complex comprising nausea
Boil	:	tender inflamed area of the skin containing pus
Bronchitis	:	inflammation of the bronchi
Bronchodilator	:	an agent that causes widening of the air passages by relaxing bronchial smooth muscle
Bubo	:	an inflammatory swelling of a lymph gland
Calculi	:	a hard pebble-like mass formed within the body, particularly in the gall bladder or anywhere in the urinary tract
Cancer	:	the abnormal and uncontrolled division of cells that then invade and destroy the surrounding tissues
Carbuncle	:	an infection of the skin and subcutaneous tissue by Staphylococcus aureus
Carminative	:	drug curing flatulence
Catarrh	:	inflammation of a mucous membrane
Cathartic	:	having the power of cleansing the bowels- purgative
Cephalagia	:	Headache
Cephalic	:	a remedy for disorders of the head
Cholera	:	a severe infectious epidemic disease due to Vibrio cholerae
Chronic bronchitis	:	the patient coughs up excessive mucus secreted by enlarged bronchial mucous glands
Conjunctivitis	:	inflammation of conjunctiva
Colic	:	a severe spasmodic griping pain

Consumption : pulmonary tuberculosis

Contraceptive : drug which prevents unwanted pregnancy

Convulsion : a violent involuntry contraction of the skeletal musculature

Cystitis : inflammation of a bladder, especially the urinary bladder

Dandruff : dead scarf-skin seperating in small scales and entangled in the hair

Deafness : partial or total loss of hearing in one or both ears

Demulcent : Soothing

Depurative : an agent that purifies the blood

Diabetes : here it refers to diabetes mellitus: a disorder of carbohydrate metabolism in which sugars in the body are not oxidized to produce energy due to lack of the pancreatic hormone-insulin. The accumulation of sugar leads to its appearance in the blood

Diaphoretic : a drug which induces perspiration

Diarrhoea : frequent bowel evacuation or the passage of abnormally soft or liquid faeces

Diptheria : a specific infectious disease caused by virulent strains of a bacillus

Diuretic : promoting the discharge of urine

Dropsy : an excessive accumulation of a clear or watery fluid in any of the tissues or cavities of the body

Dysentery : an infection of the intestinal tract causing severe diarrhoea with blood and mucus

Dysmenorrhoea : painful menstruation

Dysopia : defective vision

Dyspepsia : Indigestion

Dysuria : difficulty or pain while passing urine

Earache : pain in the ear

Eczema : a noncontagious inflammatory disease of the skin with much itching and burning

Elephantiasis : gross lymphatic oedema of the limbs leading to hypertrophy

Emetic : causing vomiting

Emollient : Softening

Epilepsy : an affection of the nervous system resulting from excessive or disordered discharge of cerebral neurons

Eruptions : the outbreak of a rash

Erysipelsa	: an inflammatory disease generally on the face marked by a bright redness of the skin
Expectorant	: aiding the secretion of the mucous membrane of the air passages & the removal of fluid by spitting
Fatigue	: mental or physical tiredness, following prolonged or intense activity
Febrifuge	: that which drives off fever
Fever	: a rise in body temperature above the normal
Fistula	: an open channel from the anus or rectum to the skin near the anus
Flatulence	: distention of stomach
Foetid	: bad-smelling, fetid
Gleet	: chronic discharge of thin mucus from the vagina
Goitre	: enlargement of the thyroid gland
Gonorrhoea	: an inflammatory disease of the urinogenital passagaes characterised by pain and discharge
Gout	: a disease of purine metabolism characterised by attacks of arthritis with an associated raised level of serum uric acid
Haematemesis	: vomitting of blood
Haematinic	: any substance which is required for the production of RBCs & its constituents
Haemoptysis	: spitting of blood
Haemorrhage	: the escape of blood from a ruptured blood vessel, externally or internally
Haemorrhagic diseases	: associated with or resulting from blood loss
Haemostatic	: Styptic
Hallucination	: a false perception of something that is not really there
Headache	: pain felt deep within the skull
Helminthiasis	: morbid state due to infestation with worms
Helminthic	: Anthelmintic, vermifugal
Hemicrania	: headache confined to one side
Hepatomegaly	: enlargement of the liver
Hiccough	: abrupt involuntary lowering of the diaphragm and closure of the sound-producing folds at the upper end of the trachea, producing a characteristic sound as the breath is drawn in
Hydrocele	: a circumscribed collection of fluid in the tunica vaginalis testis

Hydrophobia	:	exaggerated fear of water as in rabies
Hypertension	:	high arterial blood pressure
Hysteria	:	a neurotic disorder with varying symptoms
Impotency	:	inability to perform the sexual act due to failure of the reflex mechanism
Inflammation	:	the body's response to injury, which may be acute or chronic
Insecticidal	:	any agent which kills or destroys insects
Insomnia	:	-the condition a being unable to sleep/
Intermittient fever	:	a fever that rises, subsides, then returns again
Itcing	:	discomfort or irritation of the skin, prompting the sufferer to scratch or rub the affected area
Jaundice	:	a yellowing of the skin or whites of the eyes, indicating excess bilirubin(a bile pigment) in the blood
Laxative	:	a drug used to stimulate or increase the frequency of bowel evacuation, or to encourage the passage of a softer or bulkier stool
Leprosy	:	a chronic disease, caused by the bacterium Mycobacterium leprae, that affects the skin, mucous membranes, and nerves
Leucoderma	:	loss of pigments in areas of the skin, resulting in the appearance of white patches or bands
Leucoma	:	white opacity occurring in the cornea
Leucorrhoea	:	whitish or yellowish discharge of mucus from the vaginal opening
Lumbago	:	pain in lower back
Mammillitis	:	inflammation of the nipple
Menorrhagia	:	excessive or prolonged menstruation
Migrain	:	condition resulting from spasm and subsequent overdilatation of certain arteries in the brain, which causes a recurrent throbbing headache that characteristically affects one side of the head
Miscarriages	:	the expulsion or removal of an embryo or fetus from the uterus at a stage of pregnancy when it is incapable of independent survival
Mumps	:	an acute infectious disease caused by a virus
Nasitis	:	-inflammation of the nose
Nightblindness	:	the inability to see in dim light or at night
Obesity	:	an excessive accumulation of fat in the body

Oedema	:	excessive accumulation of fluid in the body tissues
Oleaginous	:	Oily
Ophthalmia	:	a term usually applied to conjunctivitis
Ophthalmopathy	:	any disease of the eye
Otalgia	:	pain in the ear
Otorrhoea	:	any discharge from the ear, commonly a purulent discharge in chronic middle ear infection
Paralysis	:	a muscle weakness that varies in its extent, its severity, and the degree of spasticity or flaccidity according to the nature of the underlying disease and its distribution in the brain, spinal cord, peripheral nerves, or muscles
Pectoral diseases	:	effective in diseases of the chest
Peptic ulcer	:	a breach in the lining(mucosa) of the digestive tract produced by digestion of the mucosa by pepsin and acid
Piles	:	enlargement of the normal spongy blood-filled cushions in the wall of the anus, usually a consequence of prolonged constipation or ocassionally, diarrhea
Pneumonia	:	a general disease in which the essential lesion is an inflammation of the spongy tissue of the lung with consolidation of the alveolar exudate
Pneumonosis	:	any lung disorder
Polyuria	:	the production of large volumes of urine, which is dilute and of a pale colour
Procreant	:	the drug which begets
Prophylactic	:	pertaining to the prevention of the development of a disease
Prurigo	:	an eruption of the skin causing severe itching
Pruritus	:	Itching
Pyorrhoea	:	disease of the tissues that support and attach the teeth-the gums, periodontal membrane, and alveolar bone
Refrigerant	:	Cooling
Remittent fever	:	a remittent fever is one in which body temperature flactuates but does not return to normal
Renal calculi	:	calculi relating to kidney
Resolvent	:	causing resolution of a tumour or swelling
Retention of urine	:	inability to pass urine, which is retained in the bladder

Revulsive : causing revulsion in drawing away of blood from a pathological area to another area

Rheumatalgia : rheumatic pain

Rheumatism : any disorder in which aches and pains affect the musclas and joints

Rheumatoid arthritis : it is the second most common form of arthritis. It typically involves the joints of the fingers, wrists, feet and ankles with later involvement of the hips, keens, shoulders and neck

Rhinitis : inflammation of the nasal mucous membrane

Ringworm : fungus infection of the skin, the scalp, or the nails

Rubefacient : reddening of the skin

Scabies : sarcoptic infestation of the human skin particularly a contagious skin disease caused by invasion of the epidermis

Sciatica : pain felt down the back and outer side of the thigh, leg, and foot

Scrofula : tuberculous cervical adenitis with or without ulceration

Scurvy : a deficiency disease due to lack of vitamin C

Sinusitis : inflammation of one or more of the mucous-membrane-lined air spaces in the facial bones that communicate with the nose

Slipdisc : a colloquial term for a prolapsed intervertebral disc

Small Pox : an acute infectious virus disease causing high fever and a rash that scars the skin

Somatalgia : pain in the body

Soporific : inducing sleep

Sore throat : pain at the back of the mouth, commonly due to bacterial or viral infection of the tonsils

Spasmolytic : a drug that relieves spasm of smooth muscle

Splenopathy : any disease of the spleen

Spermatorrhoea : the involuntary discharge of semen without orgasm

Stomachache : pain in the stomach

Stomachic : a medicine that increases the functional activity of the stomach

Stomatitis : generalised inflammation of the oral mucosa

Strangury : severe pain in the urethra referred from the base of the bladder and associated with an intense desire to pass urine

Styptic	:	having the power to arrest bleeding
Sudorific	:	an agent which induces sweating
Sun stroke	:	raised body temperature (pyrexia), absence of sweating, and eventual loss of consciousness due to failure or exhaustion of the temperature-regulating mechanism of the body
Syphilis	:	contagious venereal disease
Tetanus	:	an infective disease due to toxin of Clostridium tetani
Tuberculosis	:	an infectious disease caused by the bacillus Mycobacterium tuberculosis and characterized by the formation of nodular lesions in the tissues
Tumour	:	any abnormal swelling in or on a part of the body
Typhoid	:	an infection of the digestive system by the bacterium Salmonella typhi, causing general weakness, high fever, a rash of red spots on the chest and abdomen
Ulcers	:	a break in the skin extending to all its layers, or a break in the mucous membrane lining the alimentary tract, that fails to heal and is often accompained by inflammation
Urethrorrhoea	:	abnormal discharges from the urethra
Urticaria	:	an itchy rash resulting from the release of histamine by mast cells
Uteralgia	:	pain in the uterus
Veneral diseases	:	any disease transmitted by sexual intercourse
Verminosis	:	infestation with vermin
Vertigo	:	Dizziness
Vesical calculi	:	stone in the urinary bladder
Vomiting	:	the reflex action of ejecting the contents of the stomach through the mouth
Vulnerary	:	an agent that promotes healing of wounds
Warts	:	a circumscribed cutaneous excrescence
Whooping cough	:	an acute infectious disease, primarily of infants, caused by the bacterium Bordetella pertusis, which affects the respiratory tract
Wounds	:	a break in the structure of an organ or tissue caused by an external agent

Bibliography

Ambasta S. P. (1986) (Ed.) *The useful plants of India*. CSIR, New Delhi.

Anonymous (1948-1976). *The Wealth of India*. CSIR, New Delhi.

Anis, M., Sharma, M. P. & Iqbal, M. 2000. "Herbal ethnomedicine of the Gwalior forest division in Madhya Pradesh, India." *Pharmaceut Boil,* 38 (4): 241-253.

Ansari, A. A., Diwakar, P. G. & Dwarakan, P. (1993). "Less known edible plants of Shevoroy and Kolli-Hills." *J. Econ. Tax. Bot.* 17(1): 245.

Bhalla, N. P., Sahu, T. R., Mishra, G. P. & Dakwale, R. N. 1982. "Traditional Plant medicines of Sagar District, Madhya Pradesh, India." *J. Econ. Tax. Bot.*3: 23 – 32.

Bhalla, S., Patel, J. R. & Bhalla, N. P. 1992. "Ethnomedicinal herbal Legumes of Bundelkhand region, Madhya Pradesh." *J. Econ. Tax. Bot. Addl. Ser.* 10: 105-109.

.... 1992. "Ethnomedicinal studies on genus *Indigofera* from Bundelkhand region, Madhya Pradesh." *J. Econ. Tax. Bot. Addl. Ser.* 10: 331-332.

.... 1996. "Ethnomedicinal observation on some Asteraceae of Bundelkhand region, Madhya Pradesh," *J. Econ. Tax. Bot. Addl. Ser.,* 12: 175-178.

Bhatnagar, L. S., Singh, V. K. & Pandey, G. 1973. "Medico-botanical studies on flora of Ghatigaon forest, Gwalior, Madhya Pradesh." *J. Res. Indian Med.* 8 (2): 67-100.

Binu S., Nayar, T. S. & Pushpangadan, P. 1992. "An outline of Ethnobotanical research in India." *J. Econ. Taxon. Bot. Addl. Ser.* 10: 405-428.

Bondya, S. L., Khanna, K. K. & Singh, K. P. 2006. "Ethnomedicinal uses of leafy vegetables from the tribal folklore of Achanakmar- Amarkantak biosphere reserve (Madhya Pradesh & Chhattisgarh)." *Ethnobotany.* 18:145-148..

Brijlal & Dubey, U. P. 1992. "A survey of plant ethnomedicine of Amarkantak Plateau in Central India." *Agric. Biol. Res.* 17: 29-37.

Brij Lal, 1993. "Ethnobotany of Baigas of Madhya Pradesh – A preliminary report." *Arunachal forest news.* 11(1): 17-20.

Chaghtai, S. A., Garg, A. & Ahmad, J. 1978. "Studies on the occurence of Medicinal Plants of Euphorbiaceae from Bhopal & its neighbourhood." *Bull Ethno Medico botanical research* 3 (1): 57-64.

Chopra, R.N. Nayar, S.L. and Chopra, I.C. (1956). *Glossary of Indian Medicinal Plants.* CSIR.

Datar, R. & Vartak, V. D. (1975). "Enumeration of wild edible plants from Karnala Bird Sanctuary, Maharashtra State." *Biovigyanam.* 1: 123-129.

Datt, B. 1996. "Ethnobotanical resources of Chhatarpur district (Madhya Pradesh)." In pp 400-402. S.K. Jain (Ed). *Ethnobiology in human welfare.* Deep publications. New Delhi.

Datta, S. C. & Banerjee, A. K. (1978). "Useful weeds of West Bengal Rice fields." *Econ. Bot.* 32: 297-310.

Dahare, D. K. & Jain, A. 2010. "Ethnobotanical studies on plant resources of Tahsil Multai, district Betul, Madhya Pradesh, India." *Ethnobotanical Leaflets.* 14:694-705.

Dubey B. K. & Bahadur, F. 1966. *A study of the tribe people and tribal areas of Madhya Pradesh,* Tribal research and Development institute, Bhopal.

Dwivedi, S. N. & Singh, H. 1984. "Ethnobotany of Kols of Rewa division, Madhya Pradesh." *Proc. Natl. Sem. on Envt.* EPCO II: 34-44.

Dwivedi, S. N. & Archana Pandey 1992. "Ethnobotanical studies on wild & indigenous species of Vindhyan plateau. I. Herbaceaus flora." *J. Econ. Taxon. Bot. Addl. Ser.* 10: 143-150

Dwivedi, S. N. & Oommachan, M. 1993. "Certain ethnobotanical information of food & Medicinal Plants from Rewa division of Madhya Pradesh." *J. Indian Bot. Soc.* XVI All India Conference.

Dwivedi, S. N. 1999. "Traditional health care among tribals of Rewa district of Madhya Pradesh with special reference to conservation of endangered and vulnerable species." *J. Econ. Taxon. Bot.* 23(2): 315-320.

.... 2003. "Ethnobotanical studies and conservational strategies of wild and natural resources of Rewa district of Madhya Pradesh." In pp 233-244. Singh *et al.* (Ed). *Ethnobotany and Medicinal Plants of India and Nepal.* Vol-I. Scientific Publishers, Jodhpur.

.... 2004. "Herbal remedies among the tribals of Sidhi district of Madhya Pradesh." *J. Econ. Taxon. Bot.* 28(3): 675-687.

Dwivedi, A., Dwivedi & Dwivedi, S. N. 2008. "Folklore uses of some plants by tribals of Madhya Pradesh with special reference to their conservation." *Ethnobotanical Leaflets.* 12:763-771.

Dwivedi, S., Shrivastava, S., Dubey, D. & Kapoor, S. 2009. "Herbal remedies used in the treatment of scorpion sting and snake bite from the Malwa region of Madhya Pradesh, India." *Ethnobotanical Leaflets.* 13:326-328.

Dwivedi, A., Patel, R., Jhade, D., Sachan, R. & Argal, A. 2009. "Traditional phytotherapy used in the treatment of malaria by rural people of Bhopal, district of Madhya Pradesh, India." *Ethnobotanical Leaflets.* 13:475-479.

Ghanghat, S., & Sahu, Brajesh. 2006. "Medicinal climbers of Vidisha district." *I. J. Applied Life Sci.* 1(1): 24-25.

Ghaghat, S., Shrivastava, P. N. & Sahu, Brajesh. 2006. "Some ethnomedicinal herbs of Vidisha district of Madhya Pradesh." *I. J. Applied Life Sci.* 1(2): 53-54.

Gogte, V.V.M. Vaidya. 2000. *Ayurvedic pharmacology and Therapeutic uses of medicinal plants* (Dravyaguna Vignyan). Bhartiya Vidya Bhawan, Mumbai.

Gupta, A.K. & Tandon, N. (2004). (Edited). *Reviews on Indian Medicinal Plants.* Vol. I, II, III & IV. Indian Council of Medical Research. New Delhi.

Handa, S.S. & Kapoor, V.K. (1999). *Pharmacognosy.* Vallabh Prakashan, Delhi.

Jadhav, D. 2006a. "Ethnomedicinal plants used by Bhil tribe of Bibdod, Madhya Pradesh." *IJTK.* 5(2): 263-267.

.... 2006b. "Unreported ethnomedicinal uses of *Calotropis gigantea* (L.) R. Br. (Asclepiadaceae) among the tribals of Ratlam district, Madhya Pradesh." *Jou.of NTFPs.* 13(1): 53-54.

.... 2006c. "Plant sources used for the treatment of types of fevers by Bhil tribe of Ratlam district, Madhya Pradesh." *J. Econ. Tax. Bot.* 30(4): 909-911.

.... 2006d. "Ethnomedicinal plants used for curing skin afflictions by Bhil tribe of Ratlam district, Madhya Pradesh." *J. Econ. Tax. Bot.* 30(Supp.): 124 – 127.

.... 2007a. "Unreported Ethnomedicinal uses of *Bombax ceiba* L. among the tribals of Ratlam district (Madhya Pradesh)." *Ethnobotany.* 19 (1&2):142-143.

.... 2007b. "Ethno-medicinal plants used in the treatment of Diarrhoea and Dysentery by Bhil tribe of Ratlam district (Madhya Pradesh)." *Indian forester.* 133(8):1097-1100.

.... 2007c. *Typha elephantina* Roxb. (Typhaceae)- A wonderful wound-healer from Bhil tribe of Ratlam district (Madhya Pradesh).*Indian forester* 133(6):851-852.

.... 2007d. "Ethno-medicinal plants used by Bhil tribe of Matrunda, District Ratlam, Madhya Pradesh, India." *Bull. Of Bot. Surv. Of India* 49(1-4):203-206.

.... 2007e. "A note on some ethnomedicinal plants found effective in the treatment of typhoid used by Bhil tribe of Ratlam district (Madhya Pradesh)." *Jou.of NTFPs.* 14 (3):225-226.

.... 2007f. "Ethno-medicinal plants used in the treatment of joint diseases by Bhil tribe of Ratlam district (Madhya Pradesh)." *Jou.of NTFPs.* 14 (4):313-314.

Jadhav, D. (2008a). *Medicinal Plants of India: A Guide to Ayurvedic & Ethnomedicinal uses of Plants.* Vol.-I. Scientific Publishers, Jodhpur.

Jadhav, D. (2008b). *Medicinal Plants of India: A Guide to Ayurvedic & Ethnomedicinal uses of Plants.* Vol.-II. Scientific Publishers, Jodhpur.

.... 2008c. "Medicinal Plants of Madhya Pradesh & Chhattisgarh." *Daya Publishing House,* New Delhi.

.... 2008a. "*Enicostema littorale* Blume (Gentianaceae): A wonderful Ethnomedicinal plant against Gout, Malaria and Typhoid." *Indian forester.*134(8):1100-1102.

.... 2008b. "Unreported Ethnomedicinal uses of *Butea monosperma* (Lam.) Taub. (Papilionaceae) among the tribals of Ratlam district (Madhya Pradesh)." *Jou.of NTFPs.* 15(1):73-74.

.... 2008c. "Ethnomedicinal plants remedies for snake bite and scorpion sting among the Bhil tribe of Ratlam district (Madhya Pradesh)." *Jou.of NTFPs.* 15(2):127-128.

.... 2008d. "A Survey on Herbaceous Ethno-medicinal plants used in the treatment of various ailments prevalent in the Bhil tribe of Ratlam district (Madhya Pradesh) India." *JDRAS.*XXIX (1&2):7-14.

.... 2009a. "Ethnomedicinal plants used in leaf therapy at Ratlam district of Madhya Pradesh." *Ethnobotany.* 21 (1&2):84-90.

.... 2009b. "*Anisomeles indica* (L.) O. Kuntze (Lamiaceae): An Ethnomedicine used for the treatment of Rickets." *Jou.of NTFPs.* 16(1):75.

.... 2009c. "Ethnomedicinal plants used for dental troubles by the Bhil tribe of Ratlam district (Madhya Pradesh)." *Indian forester* 135(1):140-142.

.... 2009d. "Plants used in the treatment of various ailments by the bhil tribe of Ratlam district (Madhya Pradesh)." *J. Econ. Tax. Bot.*33 (Supp.): 59-62.

.... 2009e. "Ethno-medicinal studies on plants used in the treatment of Urino-genital diseases by Bhil tribe of Ratlam district (Madhya Pradesh)." *JDRAS.* XXX (1&2):9-18.

Jadhav, D. (2009). *Medicinal Plants of India: A Guide to Ayurvedic & Ethnomedicinal uses of Plants.* Vol.-III. Scientific Publishers, Jodhpur.

.... 2010a. "*Anisomeles indica* (L.) O. Kuntze (Lamiaceae): An Ethnomedicine used for the treatment of Peptic ulcer." *Indian forester.* 136(4):562.

.... 2010b. "Ethnomedicinal plants used as antipyretic agents among Bhil tribe of Ratlam district (Madhya Pradesh)." *Indian forester.* 136(6):843-846.

.... 2010c. "*Solanum surattense* Burm. F. (Solanaceae): An Ethnomedicine for the treatment of Dental caries." *Indian forester.* 136(7):986-989.

.... 2010d. "Ethnomedicinal plants used in the treatment of Asthma by by Bhil tribe of Ratlam district (M.P.)." In pp 85-88. P. C. Trivedi (Ed.). *Ethnic Tribes and Medicinal Plants.* Pointer Publishers, Jaipur.

.... 2010e. "Unreported ethnomedicinal plants uses of exotic weeds used by bhil tribe of Ratlam district (M.P.)." *J. Econ. Tax. Bot.* 34(4): 754-756.

.... 2011. "Weeds in tribal inhabited localities of Ratlam district (M. P.) and their ethnobotanical uses." *J. of NTFPs.* 18(1):85-90.

Jadhav, D. & Singh, V. P. 2011. Ethnobotany of Bhil Tribe: A case study among the Bhils of Ratlam district (M. P.). *Scientific Publishers*, Jodhpur.

.... 2015. "Angiospermic weeds in Ratlam district of Madhya Pradesh." *Phytotaxonomy. 15:114-117.*

.... 2017. "Floristic diversity of Angiospermic weeds in Madhya Pradesh." A review *Journal of Non-Timber Forest Products.* 24 (1):49-54.

.... 2018. "Medicinally important weed plants of Ratlam district, Madhya Pradesh, India." *Journal of Tropical Forestry.* 34(6):72-84.

Jain, A.K. & Sharma, H.O. 1990. "Certain medicinal plants used by Sahariya tribals of northern Madhya Pradesh." *Proc. Nat. Sem. Med. & Arm. Plants.* Jabalpur. 2: 155-165.

Jain, S. K. 1963 a. "Studies in Indian ethnobotany. I. Less known uses of 50 common plants from tribal areas of Madhya Pradesh." *Bull. Bot. Surv. India.*5: 223-226.

.... 1963 b. Studies in Indian ethnobotany – II. Plants used in medicine by the tribals of Madhya Pradesh. *Bull. Reg. Res. Lab. Jammu.*1: 126 128.

.... 1963c. "Observations on ehtnobotany of tribals of Madhya Pradesh," *Vanyajati* 11: 177-183.

.... and Tarafdar, C.R. 1963. "Native plant remedies for snakebite among the Adivasis of Central India." *Ind. Med. J.,* 57: 307-309.

.... 1981. "Observations on ethnobotany of the tribals of Central India." In pp 193-198. S.K. Jain (Ed) *Glimpses of Indian ethnobotany.*

.... 1991a. *Dictionary of Indian folk Medicine & ethnobotany.* Deep publication, New Delhi.

.... 1991b. "Observations on ethnobotany of the tribals of Central India." In pp. 192-198 Jain S.K. (Ed.) *Glimpses of Indian Ethnobotany.* Oxford and IBH, New Delhi.

.... 1992b. "Ethnobotanical studies of Sahariya tribals of Madhya Pradesh with special reference to Medicinal Plants." *J. Econ. Taxon. Bot.* 16: 227-232.

Jain, P. & Sahu, T. R. 1993. "An ethnobotanical study of Noradehi Sanctuary Park of Madhya Pradesh, India: Native plant remedies for scorpion sting and snake bite." *J. Econ. Tax. Bot.*17: 315 – 328.

Jain, A. K. & Sharma, H. O. 1996." Ethnobiological studies of by Sarhariya tribes of Central India." In: pp. 397-399. S.K. Jain (Ed) *Ethnobiology of human welfare.* Deep Publ., New Delhi.

Jain, S. K. 1997. "Observation on Ethnobotany of the Tribals of Central India." In pp 61-65. S. K. Jain (Ed) *Contribution to Indian Ethnobotany.*

Jain, A. K. & Patole, S. N. 2001. "Less known medicinal uses of plants among some tribal and rural communities of Pachmari forests (M. P.)." *Ethnobotany.* 13(1 & 2): 96-100.

Jain, S. K. 2002. *Bibliography of Indian Ethnobotany.* Sci. Pub. Jodhpur. 1- 144.

Jain, S. P., Singh, J. & Singh, S. C. 2003, "Rare & endangered Medicinal & Aromatic plants of Madhya Pradesh." In pp. 925-932. V. Singh & A. P. Jain (Ed.) – *Ethnobotany & Medicinal plants of India & Nepal.* Scientific Publishers, Jodhpur.

Jain, A. K., Vairale, M. G. & Singh, R. 2010. "Folklore claims on some medicinal plants used by Bheel tribe of Guna district, Madhya Pradesh." *IJTK* 9(1): 105-107.

Jain, S. P., Singh, S. C., Srivastava, S., Singh, J., Mishra, N. P. & Ptakash, A. 2010. "Hitherto unreported ethnomedicinal uses of plants of Betul district, Madhya Pradesh." *IJTK.* 9(3):522-525.

Joshi, S. G. (2007). *Medicinal Plants.* Oxford & IBH Publishing Co. Pvt. Ltd., New Delhi.

Kadel, C. & Jain, Ashok. 2008. Folklore claims on snakebite among some tribal communities of Central India. *IJTK.* 7(2):296-299.

Katewa, S. S. (2003). "Contribution of some wild food plants from forestery to the diet of tribals of Southern Rajasthan." *Indian Forester.* 129(9): 1117-1130.

Khan, S. S., Chaghtai, S.A. & Oommachan, M. 1984. "Medicinal Plants of Rubiaceae of Bhopal: An ethnobotanical study." *J. Sci. Res.* 6: 37-39.

Khan, A. A. & Khan, I. M. 1997. "Observation on certain plants used in various diseases by the tribals of Shahdol district." *Plant Sciences,* 9 (11)(Suppl.) 39-43.

Khan, A. A., Khan, S. & Singh, M. P. 2003a. "Weeds of Soyabean [*Glycine max* (L.) Merr.] and their medicinal importance in Rewa division (M. P.). In pp 245-248. Singh *et al.* (Ed.)." *Ethnobotany and Medicinal Plants of India and Nepal.* Vol-I. Sci. Publ., Jodhpur.

Khan, A. A., Verma, A. K. & Singh, M. P. 2003b. "Certain ethnobotanical informations on food and medicinal plants from Rewa division of Madhya Pradesh with special reference to rare and endangered species. In pp 249-254. Singh *et al.* (Ed.)." *Ethnobotany and Medicinal Plants of India and Nepal.* Vol-I. Sci. Publ., Jodhpur.

Khanna, K. K., Kumar, A., R. Dixit, D. & Singh, N. P. 2001. *Supplement to the Flora of Madhya Pradesh.* BSI. Calcutta.

Khare, P.K. & Khare, L. J. 2003. "Plants used in Rheumatism by Rural people of Chhatarpur district, Madhya Pradesh." In pp 301-304. J.K. Maheshwari (Ed): *Ethnobotany and Medicinal Plants of Indian Subcontinent.* Sci. Pub. Jodhpur.

Khory, J.K. (1981). *Materia medica of India & their Therapeutics,* Neeraj Publishing house, New Delhi.

Kirtikar, K.R. & Basu, B.D. (2004). *Indian medicinal plants,* Vol. I, II, III & IV (Reprint). Bishen Singh Mahendra Pal Singh, Dehradun.

Kumar, A. & Khanna, K. K. 2000. "Ethnomedicinal plants of Betul district, Madhya Pradesh." *Bull. Bot. Surv. India.* 42:109-114.

Kumar, Anand & Jagdish Lal. 2003. "Medicinal plant resources of the Kanha tiger reserve, Madhya Pradesh." In pp 255-265. Singh *et al.* (Ed.). *Ethnobotany and Medicinal Plants of India and Nepal.* Vol-I. Sci. Publ., Jodhpur.

Kumar, R., Suman, N. R. & Dash, S. S. 2004. "Traditional uses of plants by tribals of Amarkantak region, Madhya Pradesh." *IJTK.* 3(4): 383-390.

Lahri, Renu. 2007. "Ethnomedicinal survey of Sanjay National park of district Sidhi, Madhya Pradesh. India." *Flora and Fauna.* 11 (2): 289-299.

Lal B. 1993. "Ethnobotany of Baigas of Madhya Pradesh – A Preliminary survey." *Arunachal Forest News.* 11(1): 17-20.

Lindley, John. (1981). *Flora medica*, Ajay book service, New Delhi.

Mahajan, S. K. 1990. *A preliminary ethnobotanical survey in the Sirwel hills of western Madhya Pradesh.* Proc National Seminar ethnobotany of tribes of Madhya Pradesh. 14.

.... 2007. "Traditional herbal remedies among the tribes of Bijagarh of West Nimar district, Madhya Pradesh." *IJTK.* 6(2): 357-377.

Mahajan, S. K. & Pushpa Patel. 2007. "Antiasthmatic plants used by the tribals of West Nimar district of Madhya Pradesh." In pp. 190-192. T. R. Sahu (Ed.) *Indigenous knowledge: An Application.* Scientific Publishers. Jodhpur.

Maheshwari, J. K., Kalakoti, B. S. & Brijlal. 1986. "Ethnomedicine of Bhil Tribe of Jhabua district, Madhya Pradesh." *Anc. Sci. Life.*5: 255 – 261.

Maheshwari, J. K. & Dwivedi, R. P. 1988. "Ethnomedicinal plants of Bharia tribe of Patalkot valley, Chhindwara district, Madhya Pradesh." Indigenous medicinal plants symposium. 139-155. Today & Tomorrow's Printers & Publishers, New Delhi.

Maheshwari, J.K. 1990. "Recent ethnobotanical research in Madhya Pradesh," *SEB Newsletter* 9(1-3): 5.

Maheshwari, J. K. 1996. "Ethnobotanical documentation of primitive tribes of Madhya Pradesh, India." *J. E. T. B. Addl. Ser.*12: 206-213.

Masih, S.K. 1997. "Antidiabetic plants of Madhya Pradesh." *Indian J. Appl. Pure. Biol.,* 12(1): 11-14.

Mishra, D.P. & Sahu, T.R. 1984. "Euphorbiaceous plants used in medicine by the tribals of Madhya Pradesh, India." *J. Econ. Tax. Bot.*5: 791 – 794.

Mishra, B. & Vaisya, R. (2004). *Bhavaprakasa*, Vol. I & II. Chaukhambha Sanskrit Sansthan, Varanasi.

Mishra, S. 2008. "Ethnomedicinal studies of Korku tribe, with gotra names derived from plant names, from Khandwa district in Madhya Pradesh." *Ethnobotany* 20 (1 & 2): 122-127.

Mudgal, V. Khanna, K.K. & Hajra, P.K. 1997. *Flora of Madhya Pradesh.* Vol. II. BSI. Calcutta.

Oommachan, M. 1977. *The flora of Bhopal.* J. K. Jain brothers, Bhopal.

Oommachan, M., Masih, S.K. & Shrivastava, J. L. 1989. "Ethnobotanical studies in certain forest areas of Madhya Pradesh." *Trop. Forestry* 5(3): 182-196.

Oommachan, M. & S. K. Masih. 1989. "Ethnobotanical observations on certain forest plants of Jabalpur, Madhya Pradesh." *Indian J. of Applied and Pure Biology.* 4(2): 73-78

Oommachan, M. & Masih, S.K. 1991. "Ethnobotanical and conservation aspects of medicinal plants of Madhya Pradesh." *Indian J. apppl. Pure. Biol* 39: 44.

Oommachan, M. & Masih, S.K. 1993. "Ethnobotanical observations on certain plants of the tribal regions of Madhya Pradesh." *Biome* 6(1): 59-64.

Oudhia, P. & Dixit, A. (1994). "Weeds in Ambikapur region (M. P.) and their traditionally use." *Weed News.* 1(2): 19-21.

Pandey, G.S. (1969). *Bhavaprakash Nighantu* (With Commentary by Dr. K.C. Chunekar). Chowkhamba Sanskrit Sansthan, Varanasi.

Pandey, R.K. & Shrivastava, J.L. 1989. "Status survey of Indigenous Medicinal Plants wealth of Natural forest from Seoni, District of Madhya Pradesh." *Trop. Forestry* 5 (3):206-214.

Pandey, R.K., Bajpai, A.K. & Bhattacharya. 1991. "Some unique folk medicines of Baiga tribe of Mandla district of Madhya Pradesh." *J. of tropical forestry.* 7 (1): 62-66.

Pandey, R.K. and Shrivastava, J.L. 1993. Forest and tribal: An ethnobotanical observation on wild medicinal plants used by Bharia, tribes of Patalkot in Tamia forest of Madhya Pradesh. *J. of Tropical forestry.* 9, III.

Paranjpe, P. (2005). *Indian medicinal Plants: forgotten healers.* Chaukhamba Sanskrit Pratisthan, Delhi.

Printya, J.V. (1963). *The Sushruta Samhita.* Vol. I&II, Motilal Banarsidas. Delhi.

Rai, M.K. 1985. "Plants used as medicine by tribals of Chhindwara District (Madhya Pradesh)." *J. Econ. Tax. Bot.*7: 385-387.

.... 1987. "Studies on ethnomedicinal plants of Chhindwara district, Madhya Pradesh. Plants used against Rheumatism." *J. Econ. Taxon. Bot.* 11: 469-470.

.... 1988. "Ethnomedicinal Survey of Patalkot and Tamiya District-Chhindwara. Plants used against Skin diseases & Liver disorders." *J. Econ. Taxon. Bot.* 12(2): 337-339.

.........., Pandey, A. K. & Acharya, D. 2000. "Ethnomedicinal Plants used by Gond tribe of Bhanadehi, District Chhindwara, Madhya Pradesh, India." *J. of Non-Timber Forest.* 7(3/4):237-241.

Rai, R. 2002. "Ethnomedicinal studies on Bhariya tribes in Satpura plateau of Madhya Pradesh." *Agriculturists.* 13 (1 & 2):109-114.

.... 2004a. "Ethnobotanical studies in Patalkot Valley in Chhindwada district of Madhya Pradesh." *J. of Tropical Forestry, SFRI.* 20 (2):38-50.

.... 2007. "Studies on indigenous herbal remedies in cure of fever by tribals of Madhya Pradesh. In pp 177-182. Neeru Singh (Ed.)." *Tribal health.* Regional Medical Research Centre for Tribals.

.... 2008a. "Herbal medicines in cure of prevalent diseases in tribal pockets of Madhya Pradesh. In pp 175-183. P. C. Trivedi (Ed.)." *Indian Medicinal Plants.* Avishkar Publishers & distributers, Jaipur.

.... 2008b. "Herbal plants in ethnomedicinal uses by Bharia tribes in Satpura plateau of Madhya Pradesh." In pp 196-211. P. C. Trivedi (Ed.). *Indian Medicinal Plants.* Avishkar Publishers & distributers, Jaipur.

.... 2008c. "Indigenous and herbal medicines prevalent among tribal communities in Madhya Pradesh." *J. of Non-Timber Forest Products.* 15 (3):183-191.

.... 2008d. "Tribes and their indigenous knowledge on wild plants used as food and their medicinal uses in Madhya Pradesh." *J. of Non-Timber Forest Products.* 15 (4):255-263.

.... 2009. "Indigenous knowledge on medicinal plants prevalent in cure of Hepatitis among aboriginals of Hoshangabad, Madhya Pradesh." In pp 264-270. P. C. Trivedi (Ed.). *Indigenous ethnomedicinal plants.* Pointer Publishers, Jaipur.

Rama, S. & Khare P. K. 1992. "E.thnobotanical observation on some s of Panchmari hills." *J. Econ. Taxon. Bot. Addl. Ser.* 10: 97-100.

Sahu, T.R. 1982. "An ethno botanical study of Madhya Pradesh. I Plants used against various disorders and tribal women." *Ancient Sci Life* 1(3): 178-181.

Sahu, T. R., Sahu, Indra and Dakwale, R. N., 1983. Further contributions towards the Ethnobotany of Madhya Pradesh 2: Plants uses against diorrhoea and dysentery. *An. Sci. Life.* 2 (III): 169-170.

Sahu, Brajesh & Sahu, T. R. 2004. "Ethnobotanical observation on tribal areas of Vidisha district (M. P.)." *Bull. Bot. Surv. Of India.* 46(1-4): 273-279.

Sahu, B. K. 2007. "Grasses of Ethnomedicinal value in Vidisha district of Madhya Pradesh." *Jou.of NTFPs.* 14(1):71-72.

Sani, V. & Oommachan, M. 1993. "Study of certain medicinal plants used for diseases of tribal and rural women at Jabalpur & Mandla district." *Ind. J. App. & Pure Biol.* 8 (2): 83-86.

Saini, V. K. 1996. "Plants in the welfare of tribal women and children in certain areas of central India." In pp 140-144. S.K. Jain (Ed). *Ethnobiology in human welfare.* Deep pub. New Delhi.

Samvatsar, Swati. 1996. *The flora of western tribal Madhya Pradesh*. Scientific Publisher, Jodhpur.

Samvastar, S. and Diwanji, V. B. 1996. "Plants used in snake and scorpion insectbites/stings by Adibasis of Jhabua (Madhya Pradesh), India." *J. Econ. Taxon Bot. Addl Ser.,* 12: 199-200.

Samvastar, S. and Diwanji, V.B. 2000a. "Plant Sources for the treatment of Jaundice in the tribals of western Madhya Pradesh of India." *J. Ethnopharmac.*, 73(1-2): 313-316.

.... 2000b. "Plants used for rheumatism by the tribals of western Madhya Pradesh," in: J.K. Maheshwari (ed.) *Ethnobotany and Medicinal Plants of Indian Sub-Continent.* Sci. Publ. Jodhpur, 305-314.

.... 2004. "Plants used for the treatment of different types of fevers by Bhils & its sub tribes in India," *IJTK* 3: 101-104.

Saxena, H.O. 1986. *Observations on the ethnobotany of Madhya Pradesh.* Bull. Bot. Surv. India.28: 149-156.

Shah, N. C. & Singh, S. C. 1990a. "Ethno-medicobotanical studies in Madhya Pradesh, India." An Appraisal *Curr. Res. Med. & Arom. Plants (CROMAP)* 12(4): 201-217.

.... 1990b. "Hitherto unreported phytotherapeutical uses from tribal pockets of Madhya Pradesh, India." *Ethnobotany* 2: 91-95.

Sharma, R. K. and Bhagvan dash. (1976). *Charaka samhita*, Vol. I & II, Chaukhamba Sanskrit Series, Varansi, India.

Sharma, P.V. (2003). *Dravyaguna - Vijnana.* Chaukhamba bharti academy Varanasi.

Sharma, Rupa, Kantishree, De & Upadhyay, S. D. 2007. "Ethnobotanical knowledge of plants used by the rural community of Waraseoni block of Balaghat district in Madhya Pradesh." *Flora and Fauna.* 13 (2): 285-288.

Shukla, P. K. & Pandey, R. K. 1983. "Tribal life and forests: A case study of selected forest village in Dindori, Tahsil of Mandla district in Madhya Pradesh." *J Trop. For.* 9(4).

Shukla, S. & Oommachan, M. 1994. "Certain ethnobotanical observations from rural and tribal areas of Mandla & Jabalpur." *Ind. J. App. & Pure Biol.* 9(1): 41-47.

Shukla, A. N., Srivastava, S. & Rawat, A. K. S. 2010. "An ethnobotanical study of medicinal plants of Rewa district, Madhya Pradesh." IJTK 9(1):191-202.

Sikarwar, R. L. S. & Kaushik, J. P. 1992a. "Some less known medicinal uses of trees among the Sahariyas of Morena district, Madhya Pradesh." *Ethnobotany* 4 (1 & 2): 71-74.

.... 1992b. "Traditional medicine among the rural folk of Morena district, Madhya Pradesh." *Anc. Sci. of life.* 12: 274-279.

Sikarwar, R. L. S. & Maheshwari, J. K. 1992c. "Some unrecorded ethnobotanical plants from Amarkantak Plateau of Madhya Pradesh." *Bull. T. R. D. I.* 20 (1 & 2): 19-22.

Sikarwar, R. L. S. & Kaushik, J. P. 1992. "Some less known medicinal uses of trees among the Sahariyas of Morena district Madhya Pradesh. India." *Ethnobotany.* 4: 71-74.

Sikarwar, R.L.S. 1993. "Ethnogynaecological use of plants by tribals of Madhya Pradesh", *Vanyajati* 41(2): 28-31.

Sikarwar, R.L.S. & Kaushik, J.P. 1993. "Folk medicines of the Morena district, Madhya Pradesh, India." *Int J Pharmacog.* 31: 283-287.

Sikarwar, R.L.S. & Painuli, R.M. 1993. "Studies on medicinal uses of plants by the sahariya tribe of Madhya Pradesh," *Aryavaidyan* 7(1): 51-53.

Sikarwar, R.L.S. 1997. "Ethnobotany of Sahariya tribe Madhya Pradesh," India – A review. *Appl. Bot. Abstr.* 17(2): 129-140.

.... 2001. "Ethnobotany of Madhya Pradesh, India." *Applied Bot. Abst.* 21(2): 133-147.

Sikarwar, R. L. S., Pathak, B. & Jaiswal, A. 2008. "Some unique ethnomedicinal perceptions of tribal communities of Chitrakoot, Madhya Pradesh." *IJTK.* 7(4): 613-617.

Singh, N. P., Khanna, K. K., Mudgal, V. & Dixit, R. D. 2001. *Flora of Madhya Pradesh,* Vol.-III. BSI, Calcatta.

Sinha, B. K. & Dixit, R. D. 2003. "Ethnomedicinal plants sold in Omkareshwar, Madhya Pradesh." *Ethnobotany* 15: 127-128.

.... 2001. "Ethnobotanical studies on *Sarcostemma acidum* (Asclepiadaceae) from Khargoan district, Madhya Pradesh." *Ethnobotany* 13 (1 & 2):116-117.

Srivastava, R.K. 1985. "Herbal remedies used by the bhils of Madhya Pradesh." *Oriential Med.Kyoto,* Japan. 389-392.

Tiwari, D. K. & Yadav, A. 2003. "Ethnobotanical investigation of some Medicinal plants availed by Gond tribe of Naoradehi Wild Life Sanctuary, Madhya Pradesh, India." *Anthropologist.* 5(3):201-202.

Tiwari, J. P. (1981). The major winter weeds in Sagar Division of Madhya Pradesh. *Indian J. Weed Sci.* 14(1): 37-42.

Upadhyay, R. 2003 "Ethnobotanical observations on some rare. & endangered herbs of Singrauli in Madhya Pradesh." In pp 989-992. V. Singh & A. P. Jain (Ed.) – *Ethnobotany* & *Medicinal plants of India* & *Nepal.* Scientific Publishers, Jodhpur.

Wagh, V. V. & Jain, A. K. 2010. "Ethnomedicinal observations among the Bheel and Bhilala tribe of Jhabua district, Madhya Pradesh, India." *Ethnobotanical Leaflets.* 14:715-720.

Ved, D.K., Kinhal, G.A., Ravikumar, K., Karnat, M., Vijaya Sankar, R. & Indresha, J. H. 2003. *Threat assessment and management prioritization for the medicinal plants of Chhattisgarh and Madhya Pradesh (edited)*. FRLHT. Banglore.

Venugopal, K. & Raghunathan, K. 1982. (Ed.). "Medicobotanical-cum-ethnomedicinal survey of district Jhabua (Madhya Pradesh)." *Centr. Counc. Res. Ayurv. Siddha Newsletter.* 4 – 5.

Verma, D. M., Balakrishan, N. P. & Dixit, R. P. 1993. *Flora of Madhya Pradesh,* Vol.-I. BSI, Calcatta.

Verma, P., Khan, A. A. & Singh, K. K. 1995a. "Traditional phytotherapy among the Baiga tribe of Shahdol district of Madhya Pradesh, India." *Ethnobotany* 7: 69-73.

.... 1995b. "Traditional phytotherapy among Baiga tribes of Shahdol district, Madhya Pradesh, India." *Ethnobiology,* 7:69-73.

Verma, R. K. & Tewari, V. P. 2016. Some Important Medicinal Plants of Cold Desert Regions of District Kinnaur of Himachal Pradesh State in India: Their Uses and Chemical Ingredients. *J Plant Chem and Ecophysiol* 1(2): 1009.

Warrier, P. K., V. P. K. Nambiar & C. Ramankutty.1994. *Indian medicinal Plants.* Vol. I- V. oriental lonGum, Chennai.